PRAISE FOR
EVERY **BODY** MATTERS

I admire Gary for writing *Every Body Matters*. It is a book that needs to be written and read by Christians who are told that their body is a temple. I can both relate to and draw inspiration from Gary's sound words. What I found to be most powerful about *Every Body Matters* is the motivation for taking care of our body. We should do it not only for God and for ourselves but also for others. I have found in my own running that when I am training and racing with others in mind, I consistently outperform the mind-set of doing it for myself. This book gives us the tools necessary to honor God in our body.

> **Ryan Hall**, American long-distance runner
> and U.S. record holder in the half marathon

In *Every Body Matters*, Gary Thomas reminds us that the body is indeed the temple of our Lord. Gary provides a practical yet inspired approach to spiritual growth through physical fitness and reverence for our bodily temples. Those who are undisciplined in the *physical* dimension can become *physically* ill; those who are undisciplined in the *spiritual* dimension can become *spiritually* ill. Though some are born with physical limitations, others become physically weak from years of an unhealthy lifestyle. Gary Thomas practices what he preaches, body and soul.

> **Dr. Ed Young**, senior pastor,
> Second Baptist Church, Houston, Texas

EVERY BODY MATTERS

Books by Gary Thomas

Authentic Faith

Devotions for a Sacred Marriage

Devotions for Sacred Parenting

The Glorious Pursuit

Holy Available

Pure Pleasure

Sacred Influence

Sacred Marriage

Sacred Marriage Gift Edition

Sacred Parenting

Sacred Pathways

Simply Sacred

Thirsting for God

EVERY
BODY
MATTERS

Strengthening
Your Body
to Strengthen
Your Soul

GARY THOMAS

Bestselling Author of *Sacred Marriage*

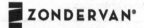

ZONDERVAN.com/
AUTHORTRACKER
follow your favorite authors

ZONDERVAN

Every Body Matters
Copyright © 2011 by Gary Thomas

This title is also available as a Zondervan ebook.
Visit www.zondervan.com/ebooks.

This title is also available in a Zondervan audio edition.
Visit www.zondervan.fm.

Requests for information should be addressed to:

Zondervan, *Grand Rapids, Michigan* 49530

Library of Congress Cataloging-in-Publication Data

Thomas, Gary (Gary Lee)
      Every body matters : strengthening your body to strengthen your soul
/ Gary Thomas.
          p.   cm.
      Includes bibliographical references.
      ISBN 978-0-310-29081-0
      1. Physical fitness — Religious aspects — Christianity. 2. Health —
Religious aspects — Christianity. I. Title. II. Title: Strengthening your body
to strengthen your soul.
BV4598.T46   2011
613.7 — dc22   2011005753

Published in association with Yates & Yates, www.yates2.com.

Cover design: Studio Gearbox
Cover photography: Getty Images®
Interior design: Beth Shagene

Printed in the United States of America

11 12 13 14 15 16 /DCI/ 19 18 17 16 15 14 13 12 11 10 9 8 7 6 5 4 3 2 1

To Bob Marvel and Torry Lingbloom,
my Bellingham running buds.
Bob, thanks for the memories
of two shared Boston marathons and one Portland,
many cups of chai tea, and fruitful times of ministry.
I respect you so much and
am grateful to call you a friend.

Torry, I'm so thankful for your friendship;
you may be one of the most pleasant men I've ever met,
but hey, it's time to get over
your frustration with a thirty-year-old rule
and join Bob and me in Boston someday!

CONTENTS

SOULS OF SILVER

"I live in a crucible between impressive success and miserable failure when it comes to personal discipline."

Mark Rhode's story is one that just about any person can relate to.

"I struggle constantly with my weight. I have a really hard time fighting against the self-defeating behavior that makes me gravitate toward sweets or fast foods. In no way do I feel like I have conquered or mastered the ability to lift up my body to what it could be. I certainly weigh more than I should—and more than I want to."

Mark is in his early fifties. He's a senior director at World Vision International; before that, he made his living working in advertising. On his last business trip, he ate twenty-four restaurant meals in a row. Like many of us, he's concerned about his health habits, and like many, he lives with a constant sense of failure that he could be doing more about his weight. He could be doing it better, could be more disciplined.

Whether you're in your twenties, thirties, or forties —or facing your fifties, sixties, seventies, or beyond— one thing is certain: you're doing it in a body, a body that not only contains a soul but *affects* your soul as well. We are not angels, pursuing God without physical covering, and if we try to pretend that we are—living as though the state of our bodies has no effect on the condition of our souls—all the proper doctrine in the world can't save us from eating away our sensitivity to God's presence or throwing away years of potential ministry if we wreck our heart's physical home.

That's the spirit out of which Mark Rhode lives. He wants to pursue God, to serve God, to know God, but he lives in a body that often seems at war with his soul.

In this, he is typical.

This book is for those Christians who, like me and Mark, recognize we might have grown a bit soft—in our bodies and in our souls. In the deepest parts of our understanding, we suspect there may even be a connection, but the application is so unpleasant that we often ignore this soft-spoken truth. For most of our lives, we have emphasized growing our souls, not always realizing that a lack of physical discipline can undercut and even erode spiritual growth.

Since focusing on the spiritual is our "default" line of thinking, let's take a few moments to look at what a healthy soul is, and then, in that context, we'll see how difficult it is to cultivate such a soul while largely ignoring our bodies.

Refined Souls

People often speak of wanting "hearts of gold," an apt and vibrant metaphor, but I suggest an additional one. Let's start speaking of "souls of silver." Silver souls speak of a divine touch, souls that have been refined, purified, and made beautiful through a difficult, sometimes brutal, refining process.

Silver is harder than gold and has the added benefit of possessing the highest thermal conductivity of any metal. Because silver is a little harder than gold, once it is pounded, it tends to hold its shape better (though such shaping takes that much more force). If our aim is to "conduct" God's presence — not to impress people on our own, but rather to be available to help connect others to God — I can't imagine a more apt "metal metaphor" to choose.

The Bible celebrates the silver-making process as a metaphor of personal refinement. Scripture assumes that we aren't what we need to be — our souls are polluted, weighted down by dross — and goes on to describe how God will treat our souls as a silversmith treats raw precious metals:

> For you, God, tested us;
>> you refined us like silver.

> You brought us into prison
> > and laid burdens on our backs.
> You let people ride over our heads;
> > *we went through fire and water,*
> > but you brought us to a place of abundance.
>
> Psalm 66:10–12, emphasis added

This speaks of a fierce but beautiful refining process that leads "to a place of abundance." To get us there, the silversmith doesn't just speak comfort and ease to his silver. He doesn't massage it into shape. No. He puts it through the fire. He even beats it and hammers it until it becomes what he has designed it to be.

The Bible declares that this is exactly what God does for his people. Consider Zechariah 13:9: "This third I will put into the fire; I will refine them like silver and test them like gold." Or Malachi 3:3: "He will sit as a refiner and purifier of silver; he will purify the Levites and refine them like gold and silver."

The refinement process is as fierce as it is necessary. The goal is to be purified and refined for God's service, just like silver:

> In a large house there are articles not only of gold and silver, but also of wood and clay; some are for special purposes and some for common use. Those who cleanse themselves from the latter *will be instruments for special purposes, made holy, useful to the Master and prepared to do any good work.*
>
> 2 Timothy 2:20–21, emphasis added

The reason I want to get in shape then, the reason I long for God's church to get in shape, is not to impress anyone, not to make others feel inferior, not to demonstrate our own personal discipline and self-control. God forbid! On the contrary, it is to become, as Paul writes, "instruments for special purposes, made holy, useful to the Master and prepared to do any good work."

Read these words again, slowly, because this teaching about the connection between physical and spiritual fitness requires that our motivation be as pure as we can make it in this fallen world. We are called to be all of the following:

- instruments for special purposes
- made holy
- useful to the Master
- prepared to do any good work

Desiring a silver soul means that we stop treating our bodies like ornaments — with all the misguided motivations often displayed by those who build their bodies out of pride and ambition — and start treating our bodies like *instruments*, vessels set apart to serve the God who fashioned them. Whether we have strong or weak bodies, healthy or sick, overnourished or undernourished, how do we begin moving from where we are now to more purposefully building bodies that function like instruments?

Dross

An athletic club I once went to displayed two chunks of silicone on top of the reception desk — one weighed five pounds, the other ten. It was a vivid way of telling us, "This is the extra weight you're carrying. Pick it up and feel its effects."

Just as our bodies can be weighted down with extra baggage, so our souls are encrusted with dross. To make silver, the silversmith has to remove the dross that clings to it. Dross is the waste or other chemical element that surrounds silver; it has to be removed in order for the silver to be refined. You don't *create* silver; you *separate* the silver through a refining process. It is an image of taking something lesser away from something greater.

Biblical writers loved using this image. Every age has its own "dross," elements that keep us from shining brightly, elements that make us less than useful, and less than prepared to do any good work. Thousands of years ago, Isaiah warned, "Your silver has become dross" (1:22).

Ezekiel prophesied, "Son of man, the people of Israel have become dross to me; all of them are the copper, tin, iron and lead left inside a furnace. They are but the dross of silver" (22:18).

The writer of wisdom explained what must take place: "Remove the dross from the silver, and a silversmith can produce a vessel" (Proverbs 25:4).

God has to remove less-precious metals from our

souls—tin, copper, lead—in order to let the silver shine in all its glory. He has to separate us from lesser things that tarnish us and keep us from conducting his presence, like using our pantry as a prayer closet. Like turning to ice cream for comfort instead of to him. Like making love to Double Stuf Oreos instead of having the difficult conversation we need to have with a loved one. Like pretending we don't have time to take care of the one body God has given us when, in reality, we're just growing soft.

This refining process will at times feel fierce and burdensome. If people aren't warned about the refining process, and its subsequent conviction, they'll either reject it as an attack from Satan or resent it as an attack from God.

We need the same attitude toward our dross as God has—a passionate desire *to get rid of it*. Consider Paul's attitude in his first letter to the Corinthians:

> Do you not know that in a race all the runners run, but only one gets the prize? Run in such a way as to get the prize. Everyone who competes in the games goes into strict training. They do it to get a crown that will not last, but we do it to get a crown that will last forever. Therefore I do not run like someone running aimlessly; I do not fight like a boxer beating the air. No, I strike a blow to my body and make it my slave so that after I have preached to others, I myself will not be disqualified for the prize.
>
> 1 Corinthians 9:24–27

Sisters and brothers, do we think God inspired Paul to write this just so that we could admire Paul and lift him up as a high, unattainable ideal properly ignored by all but the unusually holy, or so *each believer* would be inspired to adopt Paul's attitude for himself or herself?

Paul was so zealous to be made holy, useful to his master, and prepared to do any good work that he was willing to "strike a blow" to his body and make it his slave toward that end. On the surface, this does not appear to be a comforting word; we may prefer that God would say, "Don't worry. It's not necessary for you to pursue holiness. It doesn't matter if you make yourself useful or prepared to do any good work. I love you just the way you are. You *can* run aimlessly, or even not run at all; it really doesn't matter to me. I'll still love you, and you'll still be fine."

We have a total misunderstanding of grace if we think grace makes us less serious about holiness. Consider these words from Paul's letter to Titus:

> For the grace of God has appeared that offers salvation to all people. It teaches us to say "No" to ungodliness and worldly passions, and to live self-controlled, upright and godly lives in this present age, while we wait for the blessed hope — the appearing of the glory of our great God and Savior, Jesus Christ.
>
> Titus 2:11 – 13

If grace means we give up and keep on giving in to unhealthy patterns of living because it's too hard and we've failed too many times, if grace means we simply rest in God's love and don't really care whether our bodies or souls honor God, why does Paul tell the Thessalonians to "live lives worthy of God" (1 Thessalonians 2:12)? Why does he ask God to fill the Colossians with knowledge of God's will "so that you may live a life worthy of the Lord and may please him in every way: bearing fruit in every good work" (1:10)? To the Ephesians, he wrote, "I urge you to live a life worthy of the calling you have received" (4:1). To the Philippians, "Whatever happens, conduct yourselves in a manner worthy of the gospel of Christ" (1:27).

Paul wanted people to know their unconditional acceptance in Christ. But Paul also urges us to live up to the high calling of those who bear Christ's name—suggesting that effort is a fruit of grace, not its enemy (1 Corinthians 9:27; Philippians 2:12–13; 2 Peter 1:5). Being called into God's service is a glorious invitation that should captivate us and make us eager to participate. Dr. Ed Young mirrors Paul's balanced approach: "Contrary to what much of the world assumes, good works won't save anybody. But contrary to what many Christians seem to believe, good works are a primary reason why we are saved."[1]

Remember, Paul urged the young Timothy to "pursue" righteousness and godliness (1 Timothy 6:11). When you tell someone to pursue something, you're calling them to engage in an active journey. It assumes that without such a pursuit, you'll never get there. The true Christian life is a life in which holiness is a serious pursuit and a believer earnestly makes himself or herself "useful to the Master and prepared to do any good work."

For me, physical discipline is primarily about motivation. Most of us know what to do to become healthier and to be better stewards of our bodies. There are a few helpful tips we can learn, but in general, we know we need to eat less and exercise more. Furthermore, most of us generally want to be healthier. But our motivation lags.

Just as viewing my marriage through the lens of a pathway toward holiness more than happiness gave me renewed motivation to grow in union with my wife and ongoing motivation to keep pursuing deeper intimacy with her, so understanding my body as an instrument of service to God is giving me renewed motivation to take better care of it in the face of my cravings and laziness.

If we lose the image of running the race, or our zeal to do good works, we lose the motivation to be refined, to be made holy, to be prepared to do these good works. We won't be as ruthless as Paul, who said he would strike a blow to his body, if need be, to compete with all his might.

Christians who don't take their health seriously don't take their mission seriously. What we're saying by our actions is, "My life doesn't really matter." But because of the ability of God to work powerfully in any repentant sinner's life, every body *does* matter.

Tarnished

Two areas of dross that received attention in previous ages are widely ignored today: excessive eating (in all its forms) and laziness when it comes to caring for our bodies. In ancient times, these hurdles were called *gluttony* and *sloth*.

Growing up, I rarely heard any teachers talk about either of them or about how a lack of physical fitness can become a significant spiritual issue, so I never considered how giving in to them might be holding me back. It wasn't until I spotted them in the classics that I could see them in Scripture, and then it took a decade of God's gentle confrontation pointing out how my failures in both areas were negatively impacting my spirit. They weren't "damning" me, but they *were* making me less useful and less prepared to do any good work.

The last thing this book is about is obtaining some "holy" body shape. It is about having a silver *soul*, not about fitting into a certain size of jeans. Many people address physical fitness for lesser reasons — to live longer (even though their lives may lack purpose and passion), to look younger (even though they are aging by the day), to look more appealing (even though by God's providence their bodies deteriorate), to enjoy physical health (even though physically fit people die of cancer and even heart disease all the time). These are the motivations the world clings to, and while they may have some merit, there is little of lasting value in them.

The apostle Paul presents a far superior motivation

for making a serious effort to grow: to become "instruments for special purposes, made holy, useful to the Master and prepared to do any good work."

This was Paul's prayer for Timothy, and it is God's desire for us. To me, it does not sound like a heavy obligation or burdensome command; it sounds like the most wonderful life I can imagine.

It is liberation! Overeating and overindulgence lead to deprivation. Being out of shape by choice is a counterfeit form of existence. Being a better steward of your body is truly a blessing and a precious, if not literally delicious, way to live.

The Battle of the Bike

I mentioned earlier that Mark Rhode is typical in his struggle with overeating. Where he is *not* typical has to do with his passion for ultra distance events in cycling. "Ultra distance" is a polite way of saying *absolutely insane*. As I write these words, the race Mark is training for goes from Seattle to Spokane. If you've ever lived on the West Coast, you know that the most direct way to get from Seattle to Spokane is to go over the Cascade Mountains. These are not "mountains" like East Coasters call the Blue Ridge Mountains "mountains." These are mountains that make you wish you had oxygen at the top.

The race is, in fact, 284 miles long. (That's just slightly shorter than the distance between Boston and

Philadelphia but considerably longer than the journey from Washington, D.C., to New York City.)

It climbs 12,000 feet of altitude.

And the goal is to do this in a *single* day.

The fact that only thirty racers sign up assures me that there are still many sane people on this planet.

But Mark's discipline on the bike hasn't cured his propensity toward overeating or eating the wrong kinds of food, and that concerns him. It also concerns him that this is a battle he rarely hears addressed from the pulpit. He says, "We've been taught in the evangelical tradition about adultery and lying and stealing and coveting; about lust and alcoholism and smoking and drug abuse. But many evangelical pastors who preach against these things are visibly overweight or obese. I don't say this to judge them—I struggle with the same thing. But sometimes I wonder. Sure, they may have conquered the online porn, but it seems like they're 'medicating' with food; I get that, because I do the same thing."

It is this battle that has led Mark toward the ultra distance events on his bike. "For me, getting into these events is like attacking my demons head on. I choose it as a way to fight back against where I know I'm weak."

At six foot five, Mark can hide a little extra weight better than most; and since he rides often and far, he's able to get away with consuming a few extra calories now and then. But for him, the issue isn't how he looks in the mirror; it's a spiritual one. Second Corinthians 12:9 drives Mark's life and approach toward food and personal discipline: "My power is made perfect in weakness."

"This defines the whole theological underpinning for why I do endurance events. I am weak; I am broken; my sins are a lack of discipline and gluttony, among others. And riding my bike is a physical way to address what I lack, and God provides through his power."

Mark has received and lives in God's grace, but, like me, he has found that true grace doesn't kill effort; it motivates and empowers effort. And in Mark's mind, this ongoing battle — one that will never be completely won — is a good battle, a soul-forming battle, a battle worth fighting. The sobering truth is that none of us will be completely free of these struggles this side of heaven, but staying engaged in the battle will do tremendous things for our souls as well as for our physical health.

Is there any way that, like Mark, we can begin to address some neglected issues and more actively participate in God's refining process in our souls and thereby become more useful to the Master and better prepared to do more good works? Can challenges lived out in our bodies point out our need to tend more earnestly to our souls?

Our motivation isn't being accepted by God or cultivating his favor. Christ has already taken care of that. It's about wanting to run the race with intense focus, purpose, and passion.

I am not as skilled a writer as I wish I could be; for your sake, I would wish for more — more insight and clarity, and perhaps a little more wit. But if I am successful at all in this endeavor, this teaching won't be burdensome but *liberating*. What God asks us to give up are the very things that Scripture and the Christian classics testify make war against us—things that not only make us miserable but also keep us from more profound and deeper joys than we could ever have imagined—a place of "true abundance."

2

HEADS
WITHOUT BODIES

An old, popular ditty goes like this: "First comes love, then comes marriage, then comes baby in a baby carriage!" Many women will tell you that along with the baby carriage comes fifteen pounds that might take you fifteen years to lose.

Karen Yates faced the challenge of postpartum weight gain following the births of her first two children, but what really got her attention was that she also gained weight following the arrival of their third child —who came into their home via adoption.

One of the selling points for adoption is that a mom doesn't have to gain weight to get a new child, but this wasn't Karen's experience.

"It was a tough time for me spiritually, and the adoption process wasn't easy, so there was a lot of stress, which caused me to eat more."

After Karen and her husband, Curtis, finally got little Daniel from Ethiopia, Karen had to deal with the shock of caring for three young children.

"My world felt very small. I felt trapped in my own house. I took care of everyone but felt invisible. I knew I was loved, but as a young mother you pour everything into your very needy young children. I wasn't taking care of myself."

Not only was she not losing the earlier "baby weight"; she was actually adding a bit more, which made her feel even worse about herself.

Karen's spiritual diet wasn't much healthier. "You could describe it the way they describe an eating dis-order—binge and purge. One week I'd be in the Word and pray a lot, determined to get on track with God and put him first. I got up at 5:30 a.m., even if I had been up several times during the night taking care of fussy babies. But then, inevitably, somebody got the flu, chaos would ensue, and the quiet times stopped for a week."

After months of this physical and spiritual seesaw, Karen looked in the mirror and "didn't think I looked very attractive, didn't feel noticed, didn't feel very beau-tiful with Curtis. I was no longer his girlfriend; I was his frumpy wife and the mother of his kids. It's not that *he* made me feel that way; I felt it all on my own." The worse she felt, the worse she'd do with her devotions, the less initiating she'd be toward her husband, and the less energetic she became with her kids.

The element that brought Karen out of this stupor

may surprise some believers—but I won't spoil the surprise just yet. Let's look instead at why Karen's solution often isn't even considered by pastors and counselors.

Living from the Chin Up

God gave us souls—and bodies to go with them. To be fully alive, fully human, fully the people God created us to be, we have to care for our bodies, discipline them, and make them our servants in our service to God.

As I've already stated, we must guard against viewing the pursuit of God as a soul- or mind-based search in which our bodies are irrelevant at best or our enemies at worst. Though there is a long-established tradition in Christianity touting the benefits of responsible eating, there is also a tradition of those who, as one historian put it, live "from the chin up." The only part of the body they attend to is the intellect (doctrine); anything else is considered a lesser pursuit. But living from the chin up ignores the impact of our bodies on our souls.

Elton Trueblood writes the following:

> Angels ... are pure spirits without bodily needs, but men are not pure spirits. Men are combinations of body and mind and spirit, uniting in a working partnership both hand and brain. They thus have a variety of temptations and any valid religion will be frankly concerned with all of these.[1]

Swimming laps or doing Pilates won't substitute for regular study, prayer, and spiritual devotions, but taking off the shackles of laziness, overeating, and the physical debilitation brought about by ignoring our physical fitness can set our souls on a course of pursuing God with a renewed vigor, earnestness, and delight.

Christianity Today columnist Carolyn Arends writes of feeling convicted about "spiritualizing" her inclination toward avoiding physical fitness by focusing on "soul things" instead of "body things." A wake-up call provided by her parents' bout with ill health led to a significant life change, after which Carolyn concludes the following:

> Jesus called us to love God with our hearts, souls, minds, *and* strength. Just as his words disturb the comfortable and comfort the disturbed, they call the overactive to stillness and activate the overly still. They restore the soul to those who overemphasize the body, and redeem the body for those who focus only on the soul.[2]

If Karen Yates had focused only on her soul, she would have missed her "volleyball therapy."

Volleyball Therapy

The thing that initially helped lift Karen out of her downward spiral was actually very physical: "I started playing volleyball again."

At first, she felt rusty and awkward on the court. It was a bit embarrassing, having been a fairly accomplished player earlier in life, to walk into an open gym.

But she made herself do it, and the results proved dramatic.

"I noticed after a few weeks of going to the gym that being away from my kids, playing a team sport with other adults, not thinking about my duties at all, dishes, or grocery shopping—it just brought me joy. It added fun back into my life."

The volleyball playing acted like rolling a boulder down a hill—it picked up steam for other exercise in her life. Karen noticed a little more energy, a little lighter spirit, so she started going for walks in the morning with the kids. She noticed her body getting stronger and thought to herself, "I can walk a little farther today, a little faster, maybe even trot for a bit." And then those trots became minijogs and then full-fledged runs.

She started feeling even better about herself, and that gave her the motivation, energy, and initiative to become more disciplined about both what she was eating and what she was feeding her heart spiritually.

This is key. Addressing not necessarily "junk food" but certainly less than healthy food led Karen to reconsider her *spiritual* food—the television programs that weren't scandalously bad but also weren't particularly fruitful to be watching.

Because of the increased exercise, Karen also started sleeping better, which meant that she woke up with more energy and her mind was freer to pursue God.

What I love about this is that, as Karen tells her story, it's clear that mind and spirit, soul and body, began working together. Just as abuse of our bodies can gradually numb us to Christ's presence, so caring for our bodies can warm us up to his initiating grace.

The newfound energy and confidence led Karen to address her eating habits. For some well-intentioned but misguided believers, all confidence is considered inappropriate — but this is a misunderstanding of humility and, I believe, a misreading of Scripture. Humility doesn't mean an attitude of defeat; it points to recognition of dependence *and a sure hope* based on the presence of Jesus Christ. It was in large part Karen's burgeoning confidence that led her to feel happier and more energetic as a mom and become more disciplined in her spiritual devotions; it even made her "feel better sexually" — which makes perfect sense if one's body is getting into shape.

Karen warns that when women discuss body issues, they often enable each other by talking down women who are doing something about it, ascribing to them bad motives or painting them as shallow. Instead of gossiping about others, she recommends letting the physical fitness build the confidence necessary to also address other areas of life. "Most women — in fact, most people — want to be attractive to their spouses; they want to be good parents; they want to be their best. But becoming your best takes hard work and discipline. It isn't easy."

It also takes addressing soul *and* body, mind *and* heart. We can err on either end of the spectrum of neglect.

True Training

In *The Republic*, Plato recounts a scene in which Socrates tutors his student Glaucon: "Have you noticed how a lifelong devotion to exercise, to the exclusion of anything else, produces a certain type of mind? Just as a neglect of it produces another type? One type tends to be tough and uncivilized, the other soft and over-sensitive."[3]

Socrates himself was a hardy figure, a physically fit former infantry soldier in the Athenian army. He recognized that all exercise and no study creates only half a man, just as all study and no exercise also creates half a man—in this case an effeminate, soft, overly sensitive man who isn't tough enough to address real life.

It's biblically appropriate for Christians to emphasize spiritual training in godliness above physical fitness; the Bible itself does this: "For physical training is of some value, but godliness has value for all things" (1 Timothy 4:8). But to say that spiritual fitness is more important isn't to say that physical fitness doesn't matter at all, or that it has no impact on godliness and spiritual fitness. Dr. Kenneth Cooper, who popularized the word (and movement) *aerobics* argues, "A healthy, fit body is the most appropriate home for a vibrant spirit."[4]

Eighteenth-century Anglican writer William Law told us that training our bodies is essential to building lives of holiness:

Since we are neither all soul nor all body, seeing

33

none of our actions are either separately of the soul or separately of the body, seeing we have no habits but such as are produced by the actions both of our souls and bodies, it is certain that if we would arrive at habits of devotion or delight in God, we must not only meditate and exercise our souls, but we must practice and exercise our bodies to all such outward actions as are conformable to these inward tempers.[5]

This is entirely in keeping with what the Bible teaches, namely, the intimate connection between body and soul.

Body and Spirit

The apostle Paul exalts women who long to be holy "in both body and spirit" (1 Corinthians 7:34). We are not souls who can neglect our physical beings. Holiness requires a totality of experience that includes our bodies. Paul urged, "Do not let sin reign in your mortal body" (Romans 6:12). On the contrary, "Just as you used to offer yourselves as slaves to impurity and to ever-increasing wickedness, so now offer yourselves as slaves to righteousness leading to holiness" (Romans 6:19).

In fact, biblical admonitions to pursue a physical holiness suggest that even our bodies should proclaim Christ's lordship. Paul tells the Philippians that his goal is that "Christ will be exalted in my body" (Philippians

1:20). This is a prayer he has for *every* believer: "May God himself, the God of peace, sanctify you through and through. May your whole spirit, soul *and body* be kept blameless at the coming of our Lord Jesus Christ" (1 Thessalonians 5:23, emphasis added).

The sins we are to attack are not just soul-based sins — sins of the mind, sins of the heart (lustful thoughts, envy, jealousy, hatred, prejudice), or sins of disbelief — but also bodily sins: "Dear friends, let us purify ourselves from everything that contaminates *body and spirit*, perfecting holiness out of reverence for God" (2 Corinthians 7:1, emphasis added). Paul teaches, "Each of you should learn to control your own body in a way that is holy and honorable" (1 Thessalonians 4:4). In fact, Paul's definitive statement comes to the Corinthians: "Honor God with your bodies" (1 Corinthians 6:20).

The curse of today is that so many Christians equate bodily sins with sexual sins. The only possible bodily sin, in their minds, is related to lust. If they're not sinning sexually, they believe these verses don't apply to them. The contemporary age of the church is the only generation that has believed this.

We cannot be faithful believers if we ignore our bodies. Dr. Ed Young insists that caring for our bodies is a way of honoring and loving God. He brings both aspects together when he writes, "We cannot have total heart health if we focus only on the biological heart and ignore the spiritual. But true spirituality means accepting the stewardship of the physical heart God has given us as well."[6]

Silent Sermons

I asked Karen if she had ever been challenged about these issues from the pulpit, if a sermon may have encouraged her to consider pursuing her "volleyball therapy." She became silent and was reluctant to speak until I pressed her. Finally she commented, "If a large percentage of Americans are overweight, there are a lot of Christians who are overweight too, including church members *and* pastors. I doubt a sermon like that would go over well."

After pausing, she added, "People want to hear about grace and about how much God loves them, about how they're good enough just as they are. There's a lot of truth in that, but the message about weight in our churches is that it's rude to say to someone that they need to lose weight — so we just don't address it."

Sadly this is all too true, even though the failure to address weight issues can keep people imprisoned in unhealthy habits and traveling a downward spiral, the kind Karen had found herself in. Talking to Karen now, sensing the joy, noticing the strength, listening to her insights, makes you wonder why we don't want more Christians like her filling local churches and why we won't address these issues in an attitude of grace and encouragement.

Remembering her old self, Karen can recall the

shame—not just with people but with God too. It was the shame, not the confidence, that kept her from being "useful to the Master and prepared to do any good work."

It may sound strange to prescribe volleyball for what seems like spiritual ills, but it's difficult to argue when you talk to Karen. Here, indeed, is a woman who is having her soul refined. She hasn't arrived yet—none of us ever will—but she is certainly more useful to her Master and more prepared to do any good work.

And that's the promise of faithful fitness. Those of us who have the courage to address this personal issue in our own lives will experience considerable results. Improving your physical fitness will increase your overall zest for life. You'll have more energy for your marriage, for parenting, for your business.

And I also believe that being in shape means you will experience many benefits in your spiritual life. Like Karen, you may even notice improvement in sexual intimacy. Psychologically, the endorphins that follow a hard workout are an excellent way to manage stress and feel better about life in general. And I have had times of worship while exercising that are much richer than any I've known sitting in a large room singing choruses that some other writer has written.

Will You Consider This?

As I'll make even clearer later in the book, I'm not trying to get us to pick elders or deacons by how thin they are. We will soon discuss how there are different body types, and that we are called to steward only the body that God has given us, not to judge others. God alone knows whether we are honoring him with our daily choices. Seeking to maintain a particular body shape merely to please others — even other Christians — is still people pleasing. Our focus should rather be on becoming a community of worshipers who live to please God.

But for your own health and vitality, your own spirituality, your own family, and your own personal satisfaction — will you consider this? Not as a diet. Not as a fad. But as a life change, birthed as a spiritual exercise, a part of your worship, a new way of surrendering to God's presence in your life.

If I sound enthusiastic, I am. My son and I talk about this a lot, and I pointed out to him once how, though exercise and staying in shape require a lot of work and even regular pain, *not* being in shape requires its own pains and labors. If I'm going to hurt in this fallen world — and everyone of us will — I'd rather hurt and be sore getting in shape than hurt and be sore because my body isn't fit.

By God's design, we are a people with souls who desperately yearn for intimacy with God — people whose souls reside in bodies that can hinder or help this pursuit. Which will it be?

"YOUR STRENGTH WILL EQUAL YOUR DAYS"

In the summer of 2010, I was invited to join the staff of Second Baptist Church in Houston, Texas, as writer in residence. Second Baptist is a growing congregation of over 56,000 members, spread out over five campuses. The seventy-four-year-old senior pastor Dr. Ed Young has emphasized physical and spiritual fitness throughout his career. The church has an exercise club and gym on its flagship campus, and among Dr. Young's numerous books are two written with physicians (*Total Heart Health for Men* and *Total Heart Health for Women*), urging believers to pay attention to their hearts' spiritual and physical needs.

Just weeks after I started at Second, I attended the executive staff retreat. For two full days (the final day lasted twelve hours), I watched a man in his prime leading and training his staff, spontaneously teaching, praying, inspiring, challenging, and occasionally correcting groups of pastors who came in and out on a rotating basis. Watching Dr. Young in action those two days provided as much insight into ministry as completing two years of seminary education.

How thankful I am that Dr. Young's wisdom, experience, passion, and discernment haven't been lost to poor health habits. Some men and women have all but let themselves be silenced by the thousands of choices they made in their thirties, forties, and fifties about eating and exercise that caught up with them in their sixties and eclipsed the life experience they had gained. Yet here I witnessed a man in his midseventies taking the kingdom by storm. I was witnessing a picture of the prophetic words given to Asher in Deuteronomy 33:25: "Your strength will equal your days."

What Dr. Young exhibited during those two days wasn't staged with plenty of notes and anticipatory study. He didn't execute scripted teachings on ministry focus, leadership, inspiring others, holding people accountable, or helping volunteers find their calling and purpose. The entire retreat was driven by depths of wisdom and experience cultivated over fifty years of ministry. I dare say, as powerful as his ministry was in the nineties (when Second had a mere 25,000 members), Dr. Young today is an instrument of special purposes, made holy, even *more* useful to the Master, and better prepared to do any good work.

Yes, God works powerfully through the weak — and often in spite of us. His favor is not "conditional," and the rain falls on the healthy and unhealthy! But there is also a place for those who can say, as did Paul, "Follow my example, as I follow the example of Christ" (1 Corinthians 11:1). We have seen so many leaders —men and women—collapse far from the finish line. Let us learn from those few who race until the end.

What will help us get there?

A New Dimension in Discipleship

John Wimber, who wowed the church for about a decade in the 1980s with his "Signs and Wonders and Church Growth" workshops, once saw a man getting on a plane with the word *Adulterer* written on his forehead (which no one else could see). He questioned the man and found out that he was, in fact, on his way to engage in an adulterous relationship. Do I even need to point out that God rarely works this way? Most of our sins are hidden away in secret places. Few of us walk around with our sins visible on our foreheads, so when our pastors preach against them, we can put smiles on our faces and shake our neighbors' hands—and no one is the wiser.

But eating to excess and ignoring physical discipline are different. They often (though not always) show their effects only over time. Is it gluttony to have an extra scoop of ice cream if you've been working hard in the yard all day? But what about if you haven't done any yard work in a month, and that extra scoop has become a twice-daily experience?

Adultery is clear-cut; murder is absolute; stealing is stark. Excessive overeating and laziness are different in kind, and fall into the gray areas of materialism (When does a house become too big? When does a car become too expensive?) and recreation (If thirty minutes of video gaming is appropriate at the end of a school day, what about an hour and a half? Two hours?).

Though these struggles may not be black and white, they are also not without effect. If we haven't taken care of our house, our bodies, our finances, our relationships, our souls, the neglect will eventually become apparent. Proverbs talks about fields, but you could apply this to just about any aspect of human existence:

> I went past the field of a sluggard,
>   past the vineyard of someone who has no sense;
> thorns had come up everywhere,
>   the ground was covered with weeds,
>   and the stone wall was in ruins.
> I applied my heart to what I observed
>   and learned a lesson from what I saw:
> A little sleep, a little slumber,
>   a little folding of the hands to rest—
> and poverty will come on you like a thief
>   and scarcity like an armed man.
>
> Proverbs 24:30–34

Today's version might read as follows:

> I went past the body of a sluggard,
>   past the body of someone who has no sense.

His cholesterol was killing him from within;
  his high blood pressure was a tinderbox
  waiting to explode.
His breath was labored,
  and he could barely move
  without breaking into a sweat.
He said he had no time to exercise
  or to prepare healthier meals,
but he lost hours going to the doctor
  and much money buying medicines
  to treat the symptoms rather than attack the
  disease.
I applied my heart to what I observed
  and learned a lesson from what I saw:
A little sleep, a little softness,
  a life of overindulgence—
and ill health will come on you like a thief
  and frailty like an armed man.

Over time, laziness, like excessive eating, has a way of outing itself. My friend Dr. Nick Yphantides, the chief medical officer for San Diego County and author of *My Big Fat Greek Diet*, often talks about how our physical health can serve as a billboard of our spiritual health. Our weight, he says, can be a red warning light on the dashboard of our life. The problem is not the bulb itself, but rather the indication that something is happening under the hood in our not-so-silver soul. If we overeat and don't exercise, most (but not all) of us will become overweight.

Dr. David Kessler, who served as commissioner of the U.S. Food and Drug Administration under Presidents George H. W. Bush and Bill Clinton, cuts to the heart of the issue when he writes, "People get fat because they eat more than people who are lean. I know this seems obvious, but we've spent decades being confused about it ... We finally have strong evidence that weight gain is primarily due to overeating."[1]

What so many in the church *don't* see is that this physical battle has spiritual roots. Dr. Ed Young writes:

> Satan not only wants to suffocate your spiritual heart; he will do whatever he can to take away your physical heart. Jesus labeled the devil a "murderer" (John 8:44). Satan is out to cause your physical death if he possibly can. Why does Satan want you physically dead? Because it would bring an abrupt end to your loving care for others, and the whole purpose to which God has called you. With you out of the way, he has eliminated a key person God wants to use to touch your family members, your neighbors, your friends, and others in your circle of influence.[2]

Dr. Young goes on:

> How can [Satan] get rid of you? Well, he knows you're too smart to fall for the temptation to jump off a bridge, throw yourself in front of a speeding train, or drink a bottle of cyanide ... Remember: he's a con artist. He wants to trick you into doing his bidding, to cause you to think it's not too bad.

So he just might suggest more acceptable behaviors that could eventually gain him the same result, behaviors that will negatively affect your health.[3]

If this is true — and it makes sense — Satan may attempt to ruin one man's ministry by luring him into a financial trap that will ultimately become a crime and thus wreck his business and his reputation; he may attempt to ruin a woman by gradually filling her mind with thoughts of fantasy toward a coworker and thoughts of malice toward her husband so that she is weakened and enters into an immoral affair. And he may get others to eat one too many bacon cheeseburgers without any corresponding exercise, and take them out that way. He doesn't care *what* brings our ministry to an end; he just wants it to end. The latter is a more subtle attack, as the sin is not carefully defined and may not even be a sin, but it robs us of influence nonetheless.

Here's what I find sad about the church ignoring this issue: the Bible teaches that every single member of the body of Christ is essential for it to function in its full glory. *Everybody matters.* What a shame to see even *one* life wasted because every body does matter. There is no job in the kingdom so small that it doesn't matter. Every job counts. Every life is important — especially yours.

Protecting your health is the same thing as protecting the vehicle through which God wants to change the world. Is there a greater loss in this world than millions of Spirit-renewed believers digging premature graves with a knife, fork, and spoon? Dr. Yphantides likes to say, "Let's build the kingdom by shrinking the body."

Weak Beliefs

Dr. Kenneth Cooper has noted that one reason so many people fail to take care of their bodies is that "most people have a relatively weak belief in the need for good eating."[4] In other words, people say, "I know I should eat better, but ..." It's sort of like, "I know that driving five miles over the speed limit is *technically* breaking the law, but it just doesn't seem like that big of a deal, so I do it all the time."

A weak belief produces weak commitment.

Paul appeals to the highest authority to give us new motivation. If we want to develop a silver soul and become more useful to God and better prepared to do any good work he has planned for us, we will take these words to heart: "Do you not know that your bodies are temples of the Holy Spirit, who is in you, whom you have received from God? You are not your own; you were bought at a price. Therefore honor God with your bodies" (1 Corinthians 6:19–20).

We don't own our bodies; they are not ours to abuse or care for according to our own perceived wants or desires. On the contrary, not only did God create us; he paid a high price to redeem us. And when he redeemed us, he didn't just redeem our souls; he redeemed our bodies and claims them for his use as well. *Therefore honor God with your bodies.*

Do today's Christians have any sense that our bodies don't belong to us? That caring for our bodies — eating appropriately, getting sufficient exercise — isn't a matter of what we're willing to live with but is rather a matter of discipleship and obedience?

What if exercise and discipline in eating isn't as much about physical health as about honoring the God who made us?

Dr. Cooper counsels the following:

> The real difficulty is that [Christians] have never understood that their eating habits should reflect their deepest beliefs about life. In other words, they have failed to learn that the right kind of food can transform them into the energetic, healthy people they are meant to be.[5]

How we treat our bodies is a question of *stewardship* even before it is a question of health, comfort, enjoyment, or pleasure. If we're truly going to be made holy, useful to the Master, and prepared to do any good work, being more energetic and even being healthier can be essential elements of effectiveness. Many issues of disability and illness are beyond our control; they fall under the providence of God and the genes he has given us. But many issues — how often we exercise, the amount and quality of the calories we take in — are entirely a matter of choice, and these are what we are held accountable for.

The problem with the therapeutic model — eating and exercising to look good and feel better — is that everything is related to *self*: "I shouldn't overeat because it will make me less healthy." "I should exercise because I don't want to become weak and lose my breath climbing the stairs." Talking about discipleship brings God back into the picture: "I shouldn't overeat because God tells me not to, and it dishonors him as Lord when I disobey, and I want to be as strong as possible to serve him as best I can."

God's desire for us to be delivered from slavery of any kind is an expression of his love, not an attitude of divine disappointment. When we cry because we've blown it *again* and given in to yet another food-based craving, God cries with us. He hurts for us. As John Calvin writes, after redemption God treats us as a physician, not as a judge.[6] He knows it is a struggle, and he's sorry that we're feeling so awful and even that our bodies will bear the consequences of our lapses.

Dr. Young offers a warning worth heeding:

> We cannot presume that we are physically invincible just because we are Christians. If we mistreat our bodies through poor diet and lack of proper exercise, we will pay the price for it. Such irresponsible behavior may not kill us outright, but it may open the door to problems like heart disease or cancer, which will usher death into the picture before its time. And in the meantime, the enemy can disrupt and disable our lives through sickness,

which also thwarts God's purposes for us in the
world.[7]

Satisfied and Selfish

What if your soul became so refined, your heart and
mind so surrendered to God and so clearly reflecting
his glory, that your family looked up to you as a tower of
strength, someone to offer them daily reminders to seek
God, to pass on to them the wisdom of God's counsel?
What if God appointed you to serve this role, not just
to your children and grandchildren, but to your great-
grandchildren as well—but your ill health, brought
about by poor choices, took you out of this world well
before any great-grandchildren were born?

Dr. Yphantides has helped me see how selfish it can
be to callously allow ourselves to fall out of shape. If
we can't even keep up with our kids at the park, are
we truly loving them? Of course we are talking about
those who can't keep up "by choice," not those who
are saddled with disabilities or injuries beyond their
control (and I fully recognize that some hidden psy-
chological wounds can be every bit as devastating as
physical ailments). But within this framework, Dr.
Yphantides suggests, "Being unhealthy is being selfish.
Being healthy is being loving. When I weighed nearly
500 pounds I was not the only one carrying around
those 270 extra pounds. They were burdening many

others too. The joy and peace that my transformation brought have been profound."

You know why I don't climb mountains, even though part of me thinks scaling Everest would be the experience of a lifetime? You know why I'm careful when I drive? It's because there are four faces always before me who really do depend on me — financially, relationally, and otherwise (my wife and three children). There is now a church community in Houston, Texas, that has made a major investment in my ministry and cares about whether I'm available to serve them. There are churches around the world contacting me after reading a book and asking me to speak. I can't serve them without taking care of myself physically.

I only have one body and one life. By God's design, that life may end before I even complete this book. But I don't want selfishness to steal a single minute away from those I love or from those I'm called to serve.

God has given us his word and a direct command: We are not our own. We were bought at a price. Therefore we must honor God with our bodies.

HEALTHY HUMILIATION

Shortly after my first book came out in 1994, I spoke at a benefit banquet. As a new author, with great anticipation I set up my book table to sell my *one* book. I happened to be in a small town in a state that isn't known for its literacy. Or maybe my talk just bombed.

Whatever the case, I didn't sell a *single* book.

Crestfallen, I left the banquet hall feeling like a failure with no future and no hope. I drove straight to a Dairy Queen, ordered an M&M Blizzard and fries, and went back to my hotel room for some caloric therapy, after which I was dutifully convicted by God. I tried to rationalize and defend myself: "At least I'm not dealing with disappointment by looking at porn." But God wouldn't let me off that easy. Though few would call what I did scandalous, though no church would discipline me and no blog accuse me of hypocrisy,

God made it quite clear that I was using food just like some might use lust — and it was displeasing to him and destructive to me. However I might try to defend my actions as less offensive than other ways of dealing with shame, it was far from healthy for me to deal with disappointment by seeking a sugar rush and a "greasy hug" to soothe an aching soul.

That was a wake-up call — that God would even equate abusing food with lust. Unfortunately, this is a fight that often still gets the best of me. Even so, I believe that being consistently engaged in the battle instead of just giving in does many positive things for my relationship with God and others.

Now, I've since, under much happier circumstances, enjoyed numerous M&M Blizzards and probably more than my share of French fries, but I have come to discover that God does not want food or any other crutch to replace the role that he longs to have in my life. I am not legalistic when it comes to fighting this battle, but I also don't want to fall into denial.

A New Relationship

For me, a diet — something unusual or temporary — held little interest. Most people come to realize that diets can be enormously successful in the short term, but over the course of a couple of years, they almost always fail; for the most part, people gain back the weight they lose. You see this particularly when celebrities — even celebrity Christians — succeed in losing weight, write a book about their breakthrough, and then, two or three years later, look just like their pre-diet selves. Besides, most dieting books ask, "What does my body need?" While it is an entirely appropriate question, an even better one is: "What eating habits are healthiest for my soul?"

We need a new relationship with food altogether, seeing it as an aspect of life but not the reason for life. While food ultimately is fuel for our physical vessel, it is also something we accept as a pleasurable and good gift from God. There is evidence of his care for us in that his provision of food goes beyond necessity to include aspects of his generosity and kindness. But we need to remember that our use of food is something that, due to our sinful nature, can imprison us, assault us, and take years off our lives.

For me, the big change began when I saw the spiritual connection behind this thrice-daily physical practice of eating. My heart resonated with the journey of Dr. Kenneth Cooper, father of the aerobics movement, who, like me, began to steadily gain weight in his thirties and then woke up to realize the damage being caused by his neglect. What helped most weren't just the physical symptoms, however, but the spiritual imperative. Before his awakening, "it didn't dawn on me that maybe my faith *demanded* that I do my best to keep my body in good shape."[1]

What I found — and what Dr. Cooper found — was an increased sensitivity to God's presence when I began challenging my previous relationship with food.

"There is an intimate connection between the work of food in our bodies and the work of the Holy Spirit in our souls," wrote Dr. Cooper.[2]

No one would have called me fat, and few probably would have called me chubby (though by BMI standards I was slightly overweight), but I rarely said no to foods I really wanted. It wasn't just costing me physically —being more tired, having less energy, feeling a little down—it was costing me spiritually. A constantly full stomach fostered a chronically depleted soul.

It wasn't just how much I ate; it was *what* I ate. I have a pathetic, juvenile sweet tooth that embarrasses me to this day. I can easily refrain from finishing a gigantic steak or push away from the table when I know I'm full, but put me in front of a bowl of M&M's or a bag of Tootsie Roll Mini Midgees, and most seven-year-old boys will have more discipline than I do.

Early in our marriage, my young bride's appeals for me to eat better food for my health's sake weren't even close to convicting. I felt healthy; I exercised; my weight was OK. It just didn't matter to me. But as I hit my midthirties and certainly my early forties, I realized I couldn't cheat much anymore. Even more, I saw the spiritual side of this very physical issue. Dr. Cooper writes the following:

> The food you eat and the liquids you drink are a proper subject for prayer. After all, they can play a major role in your spiritual and emotional life and may be decisive in determining how well and

energetic you feel—and how effectively you are able to accomplish your daily tasks.[3]

All of us are like the aging athlete whose skills are slightly diminishing with every passing year. In our youth, we can get away with sloppy habits, but that day ends more quickly than most of us realize. And the longer it takes us to realize it, the bigger the health and illness hole we dig ourselves into. Eating habits aren't easy to break. It is far easier not to fall into such patterns in the first place. Younger readers, please take note: anyone over thirty will tell you it is far, far easier to keep weight off than to lose it.

A *Good* Struggle

Our bodies' inclination to easily gain weight actually has a positive side, spiritually speaking. Those of us who aren't naturally thin have benefits that the skinnies will never know about. Just as being bald doesn't hurt when it comes to building humility (I am humbled every time I look in the mirror), so having a body that easily packs on the pounds can foster a spiritual diligence, discipline, and vigilance that others may lack.

Japanese novelist Haruki Murakami helped me understand this insight:

> If I don't want to gain weight I have to work out hard every day, watch what I eat, and cut down on indulgences. Life can be tough, but as long as you don't stint on the effort, your metabolism

will greatly improve with these habits, and you'll end up much healthier, not to mention stronger. To a certain extent, you can even slow down the effects of aging. But people who naturally keep the weight off no matter what don't need to exercise or watch their diet in order to stay trim. There can't be many of them who would go out of their way to take these troublesome measures when they don't need to. Which is why, in many cases, their physical strength deteriorates as they age.[4]

Naturally thin people may be excessive overeaters in disguise but never come to realize the hold that food has on them. Those of us who trend toward chubby don't have this luxury; the result of our battle is clear for everyone to see. We can't get away with eating what others can eat.

God, in his providence, designed me with hair scheduled to disappear after five decades and a body that gains one pound for every time I cheat. Sometimes, it seems, one potato chip, one pound. One Pepsi, one pound. Cheese on that burger? A pound and a half.

Sound familiar to anyone?

Meanwhile, my skinny buddy not only gets extra cheese; he orders the fries and Coke and then says, "Hey, can I see the dessert menu?" One skinny friend took me out for lunch and ordered *two* entrees at the barbecue joint, explaining, "I've been trying to put on weight for the past three months."

It's so hard not to be envious!

Analyzing Our Hunger

Eventually, I found that hunger* is just a sensation — nothing more. It needn't be a tyrant. It's like lust or anger. Just because I feel lust doesn't mean I need to act on it. Just because I'm angry doesn't mean I need to raise my voice or clench my fists. And just because I'm hungry doesn't mean I need to eat.

There is a subtle and dangerous spiritual mechanism that arises when we always obey our hunger. It becomes a veritable steering wheel in Satan's hand. He can turn us in any direction he wants, and we become accustomed to letting this one sensation rule us. It affects what we eat, when we eat, and how we eat. It may take precedence over other things in our lives.

I was once (and still often am) a slave to my hunger. I obeyed it every time, because I didn't want to feel hunger. Sometimes I even anticipated it. I ate a lot in advance, because I knew I "might" become hungry if I didn't. This fear caused tension, anxiety, impatience (if someone threatened my schedule in such a way that I might not have time to eat), and the death of peace, all because I *might* become hungry.

I had to learn that hunger has a place in helping me understand my body, but I must not allow it to become an unbridled tyrant. It needs to be listened to but not

---

*Just to be clear, I'm talking about "affluent" hunger here — the hunger pangs those of us who are abundantly fed feel from time to time. I am *not* speaking of true hunger, malnutrition, and certainly not of starvation.

always obeyed. I can use reason to determine if I really need food or if I need to recalibrate my body for its new relationship with food. Hunger is a sensation, nothing more. It should never become my Lord and Master.

It comes down to this: Food is fuel. It is not Prozac on a plate or Valium in a venti Starbucks cup. Nor is it where we should turn when assaulted by stress, loneliness, anxiety, boredom, or uncertainty. It's important to know the difference between physical hunger, emotional hunger, intimacy hunger, relational hunger, and any other kind of hunger. Many, many calories are consumed in response to needs and appetites that have little or nothing to do with physical hunger but rather are consumed in response to appetites that these calories will never touch. I am not a therapist or a medical doctor and can't speak to this with any expertise, but Dr. Yphantides addresses this in his book *My Big Fat Greek Diet*.

In my own life, I had to come to a point where being fit mattered more to me than not being hungry. When I allowed myself to become hungry, over time (definitely *not* immediately), I found that I actually became hungry less often, *and in a different way*. I no longer felt like its captive.

I try to view hunger pangs in this light — as simply a sensation that takes me where I want to go (better health). These pangs are like riding a bike up a hill — unpleasant, but playing a *positive* role in my life. I have to walk through hunger pangs on occasion to get to where I want to go.

This has led to a new realm of spiritual freedom. I don't fear affluent hunger; it might not be pleasant, but it's something I can live with, and occasionally need to live with, *for spiritual reasons as much as physical.*

Benefits in the Battle

Once we engage in the battle against excessive eating, all hell will break loose — literally. It's not until we confront the subtler temptations of excessive and indulgent eating that we begin to even recognize her. She's a temptress. When coddled, she doesn't gloat; she just accepts her victories quietly as our weight increases, our waist expands, our cholesterol elevates, and our blood pressure builds — all while our souls are contracting. Overeating will take these quiet victories without even announcing her presence. She doesn't care about the credit; she just wants the results.

But tell her "no" even one time, and it's like waking up a sleeping guard dog. Enter a long-term campaign to kill her, and you'll have a sworn enemy for life.

In spite of its ferocity, this battle can produce many benefits. One of the first is a healthy humiliation. After the first month of denying myself, watching my food intake, trying to keep my exercise at a good level, I woke up, got on the scale, and discovered ...

I had gained one pound.

Are you kidding me? I wanted to scream.

There is something soul scouring about facing a struggle that you know you can't win on your own, at least not in an absolute sense. It's more than humbling; it's humiliating, and it gave me renewed empathy for those who battle any habitual sin.

Because I didn't have a lot of weight to lose, I simply couldn't cheat very often and get away with it. I could do well for most of the day, then collapse just before dinner; not gorging, but not eating well or eating the wrong (empty calorie) food. That wasted the whole day's discipline. Defeat seemed far more common than victory.

It was humiliating.

In a good way.

When you've faced defeat, you understand how others give in too. Dietrich Bonhoeffer states that when a believer takes mortification (dying to the incessant desires of the flesh) seriously, "he is more clearly aware than other men of the rebelliousness and perennial pride of the flesh, he is conscious of his sloth and self-indulgence and knows that his arrogance must be eradicated."[5]

This struggle may humiliate us, but let's be honest: Couldn't most of us use a good dose of humiliation now and then? Defeat can make us rely more on God. The imperfect nature of our struggle will at times discourage us, but discouragement can point us toward hope in Christ. It will chasten us, but chastening can make us gentler toward those who sin against us. When we're actively fighting our own sin, we will have more patience, understanding, and mercy toward others who struggle with sin. *Fighting excess and laziness hasn't led me to legalism; it has led me to deeper empathy.*

We have to get to the point where we realize that even though we value something highly, we may not be able to live up to it perfectly. The charge of hypocrisy is the dirtiest, filthiest accusation anyone can make against a Christian, but it is an unfair charge unless we preach perfectionism. I value gentleness but don't always treat others with gentleness. I value a life of fitness but don't always eat or act accordingly. I believe prayer is essential but wish I prayed more often and did a better job living in the spirit of prayer.

This increased sensitivity, sense of humiliation, and dependence on the grace of God (for we have no other hope) can make us more "holy, useful to the Master and prepared to do any good work" (2 Timothy 2:21). How useful are we to God when we live with arrogant spirits, readily condemning anyone who isn't as disciplined as we are? How holy are we when we define sin so narrowly that we live without any sense of dependence on God, mercy toward others, or personal humility?

A second spiritual benefit is that I sensed a stronger resistance to impatience, lust, and other sins. Confronting excessive, indulgent eating was almost like taking spiritual penicillin or antibiotics in that it seemed to cut the feet out from under other demands. Rather than just offer greater resistance, it seemed to erode much of the temptation.

I knew things had changed when I found myself

waiting to get out of a Wal-Mart parking lot. Getting behind the steering wheel of a car challenges my sanctification like nothing else. It was the middle of the day. I wanted to purchase one item that no other store in town had and then get out of there, but there's something about Wal-Mart — at least, *this* Wal-Mart — that resists a quick stop. The cars crawled. The shoppers' legs were moving, but the bodies seemed to be stationary, like they were exercising on treadmills. The checkout clerk chatted with every customer about every item before moving on to the next. I thought I'd qualify for AARP by the time I got out of that parking lot.

But then something curious happened.

I finally realized, *This isn't going to change* — and just relaxed.

No sweating, no glancing at my watch, no pounding the steering wheel, no running verbal commentary was going to speed up a single shopper/driver/checkout clerk/shopping-cart mover.

So I sat back, relaxed, accepted it, and tried to enjoy the moment.

Could it be that learning to live with hunger had strengthened certain spiritual muscles related to patience? At least that's what *Runner's World* contributing editor Kristin Armstrong found: "As we run we train our bodies, minds, and spirits, and our fitness levels in each category rise accordingly."[6]

In the end, I found that physical fitness offered to God, surrendered to God, pursued in cooperation with

God has enormous spiritual, emotional, and physical benefits. It is not an easy battle, but I have found it to be one well worth fighting—even though I know it is a battle I will fight, with varying degrees of success, for the rest of my life.

5

IT'S NOT
A FAIR FIGHT

Lest there be any confusion, allow me to state up front that I am not making a direct connection between being thin and being holy.

Our holiness does not rest on the shape of *our* bodies, but on the acceptable sacrifice of *Jesus'* broken and bruised body. Losing twenty pounds won't make God love you any more, and gaining twenty pounds won't make him love you any less. The glorious truth is that our skinny, chubby, overweight, and obese bodies are *all* "holy and pleasing" to God because of what *Christ* has done (Romans 12:1).

Purely from a medical perspective alone, it is foolish to make cavalier, critical judgments about others. I once met a sixty-something physician and medical school faculty member, a former college athlete who had been thin for his entire life. Following a devastating medical challenge that nearly killed him, his doctors put him on prednisone (a therapeutic steroid that treats numerous disorders) long term. If someone is on prednisone, they are going to gain weight. It's not about overeating or laziness; it's about *body chemistry*.

I've also met a woman who has battled weight issues for most of her adult life. She was very thin in her early twenties and dated a number of professional athletes, but after being raped and developing a growing awareness of long-term childhood sexual abuse by a relative, she began overeating as a defense mechanism, assuming that making herself less sexually desirable (in her mind) would deter further sexual aggression.

While the choice she made to compensate by gaining weight wasn't a healthy one (by her own admission), how hard-hearted would you have to be to expect her to *just stop it*? It's not that easy. She has been deeply wounded and is fighting the bad habits she adopted for understandable reasons. Once you've gained that much weight, your body will resist going back, so even though she began addressing what she ate, it wasn't a simple matter to regain her shape. Looking down on her, judging her, or assuming that her body shape is simply a result of laziness or spiritual weakness would be unfair and a gross injustice. She has been heroic in trying to overcome an unhealthy relationship with food, going to a weeklong intensive therapy session, joining numerous small groups, and even coming close to death after a gastric bypass operation. Implying that she isn't trying hard enough, even though she still carries considerable weight, is absurd and cruel. Her body may not show the full extent of her efforts, but it doesn't mean the effort isn't there.

Additionally, disparaging a woman who has given birth to numerous children for not being able to lose weight after the third or fourth one is to have seriously misplaced priorities. This body may not serve the interests of Victoria's Secret's marketers, but it has brought several human beings into the world—bearers of God's image, potential workers in God's kingdom—and is holy and pleasing to God for its sacred service.

There is even a potentially sinister aspect of calling people to a certain form of fitness. Princeton professor R. Marie Griffith commendably warns of the potential racial and class-oriented prejudice that can accompany calls to fit bodies. Thinness is often a "white" ideal, though, demographically, Asians tend to be far thinner than whites. Blacks, in turn, struggle with obesity more often than do whites.[1]

There can also be a class-based element in all of this. Getting fit is a lot easier if you have the means to join a health club and buy certain kinds of food, while having sufficient leisure time to take advantage of both. Judging one state (thinness) to be superior to another (obese) can support and justify class-oriented prejudices.

The last thing I want to do is judge (or encourage others to judge) people by how they look. For starters, the most brilliant spiritual writer I can think of—C. S. Lewis, who is quoted far more widely and often than any other Christian writer of the last century (for good reason)—was decidedly *not* a thin man. It would be absurd to suggest he might have had a fuller life if he had written fewer books and run more marathons or swum across the English Channel or biked his way to Scotland and back.

The reality is this: body shape isn't a fair fight. Genetically, certain races are more likely to have slender bodies, and within races, certain families run thinner than others. I'm more than sympathetic to this, as the Thomas genes trend toward chubby.

The church is to be a healing place of grace, calling all of us from glory to glory, not a hard-edged place of condemnation and judgment. Over thirty years ago, one critical comment by a concert reviewer set the singer Karen Carpenter on a course that led to a fatal bout with anorexia. She was so young and talented, with a near-hypnotic voice, that her early demise was all the more tragic. Given this reality, we must be careful to avoid speaking out indiscriminately and critically about weight, knowing that in the wrong context, we may launch a young person on a battle that could literally end her life. Let's also be sympathetic to people who live in a culture that feeds and targets our appetites.

Three Feasts a Day

Most contemporary believers living in affluent countries must ever exist on the precipice of *some* form of gluttony, in large part because never has a society seemed so skillful at producing obesity.[2] Keep in mind, the most common daily *lunch* in North America — some kind of meat, vegetables, and drink, maybe even a dessert — constituted a *feast* in Old Testament times. And we're not even talking about our day-to-day dinners! Our expectations for a certain kind and quantity and variety of food — two or three times a day — are wildly out of scale with biblical realities and ancient warnings.

Dr. David Kessler's study of overeating in America showed that food producers have found just the right mixture of fat, sugar, and salt to all but addict us to certain kinds of foods. And they have engineered food that barely needs to be chewed so we can wolf it down fast and keep piling it in, which makes the process of eating even more enjoyable. "When you're eating these things," one researcher commented, "you've had 500, 600, 800, 900 calories before you know it." Kessler's conclusion explains why we can gorge ourselves almost without thinking: "Refined food simply melts in the mouth."[3]

What makes the battle against overeating and obesity so difficult is that companies have a financial interest in finding the perfect combination of taste, ease of eating, meltdown of the food, and what researchers call "the early hit" (the immediate sensation you get when the food enters your mouth). Food producers actively manipulate all of these elements to increase the demand for their product.

So if you feel like you're being targeted, you are.

One venture capitalist bluntly confessed, "The goal is to get you hooked."[4] They've even found a way to engineer food that literally changes the way we feel. Kessler states, "Highly rewarding food becomes reinforcing because we've learned that it makes us feel better, motivating us to return."[5]

Here is what you and I are up against, and it explains why it is so difficult to change the way we eat:

> When our brain circuits have adapted to a predictable pattern of behavior, we find ourselves in a cycle of cue-urge-reward-habit. We repeat the same action over and over because that's what we've become accustomed to doing ... At that point, we are almost literally thoughtless.[6]

The cue — seeing the food on a TV commercial or pictured perfectly prepared in a magazine — leads to the urge: "I gotta have that!" We give in and are immediately rewarded for doing so: "This tastes incredible! I feel so good right now." Follow that through just a couple times, and suddenly we have a *habit*. The initial cue has become a slavish demand and eventually can even ripen into an addiction.

If the church doesn't consciously warn fellow members of what is going on, arming them with biblical and practical knowledge, we are letting fellow members of the kingdom be picked off by companies that profit from our misery, whose very goal is to get us to thoughtlessly consume products that are harmful to our bodies, souls, witness, and health.

A fascinating study published in the April 2010 issue of *International Journal of Obesity* examined historical paintings of the Last Supper throughout the centuries. Since the Last Supper is a major moment in Christian history, painters in every age left behind their own interpretations. By comparing the size of the disciples' heads and bodies to the food on the table, these researchers were able to reach some remarkable conclusions: between the years 1000 and 2000, the main course size pictured on the table in front of Jesus and his disciples increased by 69 percent, plate size by 66 percent, and the loaves of bread by 23 percent. The greatest increase in size came after 1500.[7]

The biblical account mentions just bread and wine, but later paintings add fish, lamb, pork, and other delicacies. As we've grown in affluence, we've come to expect certain types of meals, without even thinking about it or evaluating it. Painters aren't purposefully choosing to create larger dishes; they're simply making assumptions based on their contemporary experience, and for the last several centuries, these assumptions keep getting larger and larger.

My daughter befriended an exchange student from the Netherlands who told me that one of the biggest surprises for her coming to the United States was the size of our plates and the portions that we eat at virtually every meal.

All of this means that good health will require us to confront and resist the physical, spiritual, and cultural enticements that war against us.

End Product

What our body is today speaks primarily of our past—hundreds of thousands, if not millions, of decisions about what we ate and whether we exercised—but not knowing your past, none of us should judge you or praise you. We don't know the battles you've faced, nor do we know if you come from a freakishly thin family that allows you to eat whatever you want, with no exercise, without ever gaining a pound, or whether you come from a genetic makeup that will punish you for eating a single saltine cracker.

What we *can* control is where we're going. If we've been less than healthy, we can commit ourselves, as a spiritual exercise, to deal with the *spiritual* issues behind the *physical* problem. An obviously overweight person, honoring God on any given day by being responsible in eating and exercise, is moving *toward* God, and that pleases him, while a thin person eating whatever he wants may not even realize the damage he is doing to his soul as he eats away any sensitivity to God's presence.

Our battle is *today*. Because of God's grace, yesterday doesn't count. Because of God's hope, worry about tomorrow is inappropriate. *This* moment, *this* day, *this* hour, are we being faithful toward God, honoring him with what we eat and don't eat, and taking care of our bodies accordingly?

This means there is much hope for leaders or parents who are out of shape. Because we embrace a gospel of grace and forgiveness, a person's past doesn't disqualify her from service in the future (and aren't we glad this is true?). A pastor or parent may say, "I have to admit that God has convicted me that this is an area in my life in which I haven't been as faithful as I'd like to be. Let's face this together."

Such a person can then become a leader, modeling conviction, repentance, and reliance on the Holy Spirit for personal transformation. In some ways, such a leader will even have an advantage, as his or her progress will be much more visible than someone who is already looking trim and fit. Whenever a child, employee, or church member faces a struggle in the future, they can look at their leader's transformed self and say, "God changed him; God changed her—and he can change me too."

If any leader will take this seriously and begin to experience for herself or himself the benefits I'm talking about, they will likely become an enthusiastic proponent of spiritual and physical fitness. I've seen this happen often. The results are quite amazing.

If we remember that humility is the chief virtue —if we look at fitness through the lens of humility and build community that embraces humility—then we can look at this issue through the lens of encouragement instead of judgment, inspiration instead of condemnation.

6

IS BEING OVERWEIGHT A SIN?

The approximate value of a single M&M is less than a penny. The approximate value of a three-year-old Honda CRV is about $20,000.

I came *this close* to one of the most foolish misplaced priorities in my life.

In order to set the stage, I confess that I have the taste buds of a seven-year-old boy. You might think in my forties I would have lost my sweet tooth, but in reality few things make me as happy as a box of Hot Tamales or a bag of M&Ms.

On one occasion, I was driving on the freeway, popping some M&Ms into my mouth when one slipped away and fell onto the floorboard. I all but forgot I was driving in my frantic determination to get that penny piece of candy back into my hand.

Have you ever swerved while driving only to realize just how stupidly you're acting? I was literally risking not just $20,000 worth of machinery but my own life (and perhaps someone else's), all for a tiny dot of sugar-coated chocolate.

Whether or not this episode constituted a "sin," it was extremely foolish and even reckless. It certainly wasn't wise.

In the same vein, I believe it is most helpful to use the language of "wisdom" and "stewardship" when talking about care of the body. But I know some readers are thinking, "Man up, Gary, and answer the question: Is being overweight a sin?"

To answer the question of whether being overweight is a sin, we have to look at the biblical evidence. From the ancients' (the Christian classics) numerous denunciations of gluttony, I assumed I could pick from among two or three dozen verses that scathingly and clearly denounce gluttony or excessive and indulgent eating. In reality, the Bible doesn't say a lot about gluttony. There are a few direct references and several indirect ones, but not as many as I expected to find.

The Biblical Witness

One of the seemingly clearest verses denouncing gluttony is Philippians 3:19: "Their destiny is destruction, their god is their stomach, and their glory is in their shame. Their mind is set on earthly things." The challenge with this verse is that *koilia* (stomach) is a generic term in the Greek that can refer to the actual stomach but also to bodily desires in general. So while it clearly *could* apply to food, it doesn't necessarily do this, at least not exclusively.

Proverbs 23:19–21 provides the clearest warning:

> Listen, my son, and be wise,
>   and set your heart on the right path:
> Do not join those who drink too much wine
>   or gorge themselves on meat,
>   for drunkards and gluttons become poor,
>   and drowsiness clothes them in rags.

This is a clear and direct denunciation of overindulgence in eating and drinking, but even here, the implication is not necessarily that excessive eating and drinking is unhealthy in itself but that it may lead to poverty.

Proverbs 23:2 advises to "put a knife to your throat if you are given to gluttony," particularly in the home of a powerful man, but in context this speaks as much about demonstrating discipline in front of someone who could hire or fire you than it does gluttony or indulgence. It is more about social awareness than about healthy eating.

Proverbs 25:27 warns against becoming overly fond of sweets: "It is not good to eat too much honey," laying down the principle that the *quantity* of a good thing can become a bad thing. "If you find honey, eat just enough—too much of it, and you will vomit" (25:16).

The writer of Ecclesiastes warns of the insatiable

aspect of gluttony and excessive eating: "Everyone's toil is for their mouth, yet their appetite is never satisfied" (6:7). And Solomon states that it is a disgrace to one's father to be "a companion of gluttons" (Proverbs 28:7).

That's the extent of the Old Testament teaching. Keep in mind that most of the Old Testament teaching on gluttony derives from Wisdom literature, which any first-year seminarian can tell you cannot be treated in the same manner as, for instance, the Ten Commandments or the direct teachings of Jesus. While Wisdom literature is every bit as inspired as the other Scriptures, its intent is to offer general principles, not laws, and it must be read accordingly.

In the New Testament, Paul indirectly addresses gluttony and overeating in his first letter to the Corinthians: "So whether you eat or drink or whatever you do, do it all for the glory of God" (10:31). I say *indirectly* because Paul is primarily talking about whether it is lawful to eat food offered to idols; he isn't specifically addressing self-discipline. Earlier in this same letter, he writes, "'Food for the stomach and the stomach for food, and God will destroy them both'" (6:13). However, this statement comes in the middle of an argument against sexual immorality, and Paul is likely responding to one of the Corinthians' own quotes. Paul is emphatic in this verse, however, that our bodies are for the Lord and not for us to abuse.

In another indirect example, Paul describes the Cretans as "lazy gluttons" and declares that they should be rebuked sharply (Titus 1:12–13). At the very least, we can safely say that Paul was not a fan of those who overindulged with food.

That's about it. Clearly, the Bible looks with disfavor on gluttony and indulgence but doesn't denounce it as consistently or as directly as it denounces sexual sin, laziness, idolatry, materialism, and many other social ills. It's a fair assessment to state that the biblical witness warns us about gluttony and indulgence, but the teaching is relatively brief and somewhat indirect.

Keep in mind that for much of the period during which Scripture was written, people fought against starvation. They did not live in a land with the kind of food, and certainly not the abundance of food, that we enjoy today. It would have looked foolish to warn a people who lived in a time of famine and scarcity not to overeat. I suspect Paul would more directly address overeating if he were writing his epistles today, but this is speculation — and with the oblique warnings that exist in Scripture, I think it is *fair* speculation. On the other hand, we must trust God's providence that his Word contains all the moral instruction that is vital for the health of our souls. We don't want to do what the Pharisees did — create new "laws" based on scriptural principles.

Given this, I believe it is reasonable for the church to focus on sexual immorality and lack of empathy toward the poor (materialism) over gluttony and a lack of physical fitness. We may err in our silence on one issue, but at least we're silent on the issue with which Scripture has less to say.

Therefore, I don't believe it's appropriate to say that being overweight is a sin. For starters, is being an alcoholic a sin? Of course not! But getting drunk is. Consistently gorging on food could, indeed, be considered sinful, but the state of carrying too much weight might not be due to this, and it would be misleading and unkind to categorically declare it a sin to be overweight. Besides, what constitutes being overweight? The Body Mass Index (BMI) isn't found in Scripture. I will summarize it this way: *Sin can lead us to become overweight, but being overweight is not, in and of itself, a sin.*

However, in the history of Christian spirituality, gluttony and indulgence receive an abundance of attention, and we would be foolish to ignore it. If Jack Nicklaus, Tiger Woods, Arnold Palmer, and Sam Snead all gave me the same advice about how to improve my golf swing, it would be silly to persist in my bad form. When so many of the writers of the Christian classics tell us to "be careful" with gluttony, we would be wise to pay heed.

The Ancient Witness

The early church father Chrysostom set the stage when he warned, "The god of the belly overwhelms the whole body. Set self-constraint as a bound to it as God sets the sand to the sea."[1] On another occasion, Chrysostom is even stronger:

The body was not made for the purpose of fornication, nor was it created for gluttony. It was meant
to have Christ as its head, so that it might follow
him. We should be overcome with shame and
horror-struck if we defile ourselves with such great
evils."[2] Jerome (a contemporary of Chrysostom)
added, "The eating of flesh, and drinking of wine,
and fullness of stomach, is the seed-plot of lust.[3]

The ancients believed gluttony and sloth weaken
us and make us more vulnerable against other sins,
particularly lust. John Climacus, who wrote the most
widely used guidebook for ascetics* in the seventh century, *The Ladder of Divine Ascent*, called gluttony "the
prince of the passions," and the belly "the cause of all
human shipwreck."[4] One of the great dangers of gluttony, in John's view, was that "to be unfaithful in the
small things is to be unfaithful in the great, and this
is very hard to bring under control."[5] He adds, "Many
who keep a hard check on the stomach can more easily
restrain the blathering tongue."[6] To put a contemporary spin on it, if you can't control yourself at the buffet, you'll likely be massacred when facing the sins of
power, gossip, or ambition.

John Climacus agrees with Jerome in seeing a special connection between gluttony and lust: "The man

---

*The word *ascetic* has a root meaning of discipline, training, and
exercise. Asceticism stressed strict living in solitude or small
groups, usually devoted to prayer, meditation, and poverty. It
was a simple life of abstinence, fasting, and obedience.

who looks after his belly and at the same time hopes to control the spirit of fornication is like someone trying to put out a fire with oil."[7] That's a valuable lesson. Lust can be attacked indirectly by addressing other weaknesses that diminish our overall self-control.

This connectedness of vices is a lesson that today's church needs to recapture. Just as growing in one virtue helps us in all aspects of character, so one compromise endangers everything. A dike needs just one hole to make whatever it is protecting vulnerable to the flood. It doesn't matter if the "hole" is pride, gluttony, lust, ambition, bitterness, or jealousy; a pampered vice produces many offspring.

François Fénelon* warns, "But the most dangerous thing is that the soul, by the neglect of little things, becomes accustomed to unfaithfulness."[8] This is such an important phrase that I want to repeat it to make sure you get the point: *"The soul, by the neglect of little things, becomes accustomed to unfaithfulness."*

There is no doubt that today's church views gluttony as a relatively "little thing." Our silence on the subject is more than enough evidence to suggest this. But "little things" can do great harm if they make us accustomed to unfaithfulness.

How subtle temptation can be, that our hearts only gradually grow callous, in an almost imperceptible way, as we ignore the steady erosion of our heart's godly pas-

---

*Eighteenth-century author of the renowned classic *Christian Perfection*.

sions in the face of the unrelenting force of gluttony. The real question is, are my eating habits slowly pulling me away from an intimate walk with God? Is food serving me by providing necessary nutrition, or is it holding me back by gradually making me increasingly insensitive to God's voice and presence? Is food shaping me into a man who lives solely for his own gratification rather than nourishing me to look after the needs of others?

In *The Cost of Discipleship*, Dietrich Bonhoeffer made this comment:

> Strict exercise of self-control is an essential feature of the Christian's life ... Fasting helps to discipline the self-indulgent and slothful will which is so reluctant to serve the Lord, and it helps to humiliate and chasten the flesh ... If there is no element of asceticism in our lives, if we give free rein to the desires of the flesh, ... we shall find it hard to train for the service of Christ."[9]

Dull Souls

In his book *A Serious Call to a Devout and Holy Life*, William Law issued this warning:

> A person that eats and drinks too much does not feel such effects from it as those do who live in notorious instances of gluttony and intemperance; but yet his course of indulgence, though it be not scandalous in the eyes of the world nor such as

torments his own conscience, is a great and constant hindrance to his improvement in virtue; it gives him eyes that see not and ears that hear not; it creates a sensuality in the soul, increases the power of bodily passions, and makes him incapable of entering into the true spirit of religion.[10]

Instead of attacking our anger or lust head-on, John Climacus suggests going to war with gluttony: "If, in your humility, you reduce the amount you eat, your passions will be correspondingly reduced. To have an insensitive heart is to be dulled in mind, and food in abundance dries up the well of tears."[11]

By "well of tears," Climacus is referring to a humble, repentant attitude toward God, recognizing our need for him and living in a state of repentance — something we moderns aren't exactly known for. I can't explain why but I know from experience that when I am being disciplined around food, I am more mindful of God. When I am charging from buffet to buffet — a full breakfast to a hearty lunch to a lavish dinner — it is hard to remain aware of and sensitive to his presence.

I am no model for extended fasting. One of the challenges is that such fasts wear me out and keep me from doing just about anything else. If you have this experience too, you may, like me, find that what I call "spot fasting" — from certain foods or meals, or at certain times — is more helpful. Such fasts can be an even greater challenge in that they address our eating habits every day, not just once a week or once a month.

You can "spot fast" from breakfast to dinner, or even lunch to dinner, or dinner to breakfast. This may sound pitifully anemic to those who practice a more heroic form of fasting, but keep in mind that some studies have shown that snacking is the downfall of many Americans. France has a cultural norm of eating only during certain times of the day, which provides a built-in safeguard against overeating—and so generally we find that French people are thinner. North Americans tend to snack a lot between meals and usually fail to adjust the overall calorie count accordingly. That's why I'm a big fan of spot fasting. When you finish dinner, for instance, floss and brush your teeth and say, "That's it until morning." This act keeps me from eating for another twelve hours, thereby reducing my season of temptation by half. Even better, I am set free to focus on serving God. With my nutritional needs for the day met, I can focus on other things.

Ancient Attention

Heroic fasting and iron-willed discipline, all done for the sake of piety instead of purpose, leads to the dead end of condemnation and guilt. John Calvin appropriately, and I believe wisely, challenged both the ultra-asceticism of John Climacus in the Eastern Orthodox tradition and what he called the "superstition" of the Roman Catholic tradition (which saw heroic fasting as earning merit on its own), but he still upheld the value of reasonable and limited fasting for spiritual health. I've read, but haven't been able to verify, that Calvin ate just one meal a day. Some of Calvin's followers, unfortunately, focused more on his denunciations of superstitious fasting and ignored his writings about healthy abstinence.

Two centuries later, John Wesley was a tireless advocate of responsible eating, as was the English evangelist George Whitefield. In fact, Wesley's book on responsible eating (*Primitive Physick*) became one of the best-selling medical books in the late eighteenth century.[12]

Wesley's words of advice in one of his sermons are helpful:

> Many of those who now fear God are deeply sensible how often they have sinned against him by the abuse of these lawful things. They know how much they have sinned by excess of food; how long they have transgressed the holy law of God with regard to temperance, if not sobriety too; how they have indulged their sensual appetites, perhaps to the impairing even their bodily health, certainly to the no small hurt of their soul ... To remove therefore the effect, they remove the cause; they keep at a distance from all excess. They abstain, as far as is possible, from what had well nigh plunged them in everlasting perdition. They often wholly refrain; always take care to be sparing and temperate in all things.[13]

Wesley's conclusion that overeating goes beyond bodily health "to the no small hurt of their soul" sums up a healthy, balanced, classical view of the danger of overeating. Centuries of Christian thinkers have testified to the negative spiritual consequences of gluttony.

Henry Drummond worked with students during the dawn of a new scholasticism and scientific discovery in the late nineteenth century. He found fame by applying his impeccable logic to spiritual matters:

> If you would know God's will in the higher [realm], therefore, you must begin with God's will in the lower: which simply means this — that if you want to live the ideal life, you must begin with the ideal body. The law of moderation, the law of sleep, the law of regularity, the law of exercise, the law of cleanliness — this is the law or will of God for you. This is the first law, the beginning of His will for you.[14]

Drummond told young men and women that if they truly want to know God's will for their lives, it will begin with what they put in their bodies and the care they take to stay in shape. It's no good asking God what country you should serve in if the body you will serve with is being abused by neglect or a voracious, unchecked appetite.

Drummond goes on:

> Whoever heard of gluttony doing God's will, or laziness, or uncleanness, or the man who was

careless and wanton of natural life? Let a man disobey God in these, and you have no certainty that he has any true principle for obeying God in anything else: for God's will does not only run into the church and the prayer-meeting and the higher chambers of the soul, but into the common rooms at home down to the wardrobe and larder and cellar, and into the bodily frame down to blood and muscle and brain.[15]

As one who has spoken at numerous college chapels, I frequently hear the impassioned plea, "What is God's will for my life?"

Drummond's first response might be, "Get in shape."

Granted, the classics are not Scripture. They must be tested, discussed, and occasionally set aside. But when so many throughout all ages of the church testify so clearly, passionately, and exhaustively about the spiritual dangers of overeating, we would be wise to pay attention.

So I go to war against gluttony and indulgence, not because I want God to love me more, but because God, who already loves me perfectly, warns me that gluttony and excess are my enemies — regardless of how good they may sometimes feel. I go to war against gluttony, not to build a body that others admire, but to maintain a soul "prepared to do any good work" that God can use to bless others. I go to war against gluttony because those who have walked closely with God warn me that overeating dulls me to God's accepting presence, makes me more vulnerable to other sins, negatively affects my relationships with other people, and robs me of the joy rightfully mine as an adopted, deeply loved, and accepted child of God.

SOCIALLY CONTAGIOUS

Pro Athletes Outreach regularly invites me to speak at private conferences of professional athletes and coaches. One conference addressed the needs of football players and their families. I walked into the out-of-the-way resort weighing in at 165 pounds but still trying to lose a few more before an upcoming race. When an offensive linemen, whose arms were literally bigger than my thighs, walked by, my wife pleaded with me, "Gary, please don't mention the fact that you're trying to lose weight. These guys will lose all respect for you."

She had a point. The ground *shook* when these guys ran. The city of Boston would be repairing potholes for weeks if these guys took part in the marathon. When you see professional football players together on the field, surrounded only by each other, you don't realize just how big and strong these men are.

Three months later, I found myself in Duluth, Minnesota, to run in the Grandma's Marathon — a large marathon with a strong history, a fast course, and a purse for the winners — which means it draws elite Kenyan runners.

I stayed at the same hotel as some of the Kenyans, and on one occasion I shared an elevator ride with one — a man about my height but who must have weighed twenty-five to thirty pounds less than I did. As the runner moved off the elevator with all the grace of an athlete trained to excel, I looked at myself and said, "Dude, you gotta start passing up the burgers and start eating more salads."

In one situation, I felt ridiculously small and thin; in the other, I felt a bit heavy, lax, and undisciplined, even though my weight was identical in both situations. The *same body* created two entirely different impressions. The environment I was in made me look at myself differently.

My experience was actually the subject of research in a study published in the *New England Journal of Medicine*, which found that obesity is "socially contagious." Your social environment has a tremendous impact on your own journey of either gaining or losing weight. When your close friends, spouse, or siblings slowly gain weight, you are likely to follow, and the reverse appears to be true as well: when those around you lose weight, you are much more likely to be motivated to lose weight yourself.[1]

Perhaps this is what has happened with Christians.

When everyone around us is just a little bit heavier than we are and exercises a little less, we think we're doing fine — regardless of our true condition — and aren't as motivated to make a change.

Since the contemporary church tends to define sinful indulgence as anything having to do with sexual immorality or illicit substances (getting drunk or stoned), we're acutely sensitive to avoid such sins. But many of us feel quite comfortable with bodies that don't honor God — in large part because everyone else in our church looks just like us. Too many of us are members of Calorie Chapel!

Perhaps this is why the Bible consistently speaks of the pursuit of holiness in a corporate context (the church) rather than as individual efforts. "In him the whole building is joined together and rises to become a holy temple in the Lord. And in him you too are being built together to become a dwelling in which God lives by his Spirit" (Ephesians 2:21–22).

Painting Shackles

As a Christian physician, Dr. Scott VanLue became convinced that he needed to stop simply treating the symptoms and start addressing the underlying problems in his patients' lives. After nearly a decade of practicing traditional medicine, in which he saw thirty to forty patients a day, Scott came to the conclusion, "I'm not really helping anybody here; I'm just giving out meds."

He sold his practice and opened a clinic that focuses on wellness. "I love physiology. I love helping people by going back to the basics. Instead of just treating hypertension with drugs, I could treat the visceral fat that *causes* hypertension, and sometimes I can get people off medicine within weeks."

One thing that particularly grieves him is seeing people gradually grow comfortable with their poor state of health, even when they can do something about it. It's one thing for a person who loses a limb to learn how to accommodate that loss, but Scott finds too many people suffering from the effects of obesity who gradually accept their state, take drugs to treat the worst symptoms (high blood pressure, etc.), and do virtually nothing to address the cause.

My own physician recently told me of a patient who was, among other things, considerably overweight and still gaining. Every statistical indicator of health was getting steadily worse. My doctor told him, "You need to get serious about losing some weight. You need to stop smoking, and it wouldn't hurt to cut down on the drinking."

The man replied, "But doctor, I've got to have my nightly cigar and bowl of ice cream, and what's an evening without a nightcap?"

The doctor replied, "Then you need to prepare to die, and you should ask yourself, Are those things more important to me than future years? — because that's the trade you're making."

Because we don't *suddenly* gain fifty pounds, we

gradually grow used to the decreased mobility, the slow onset of breathlessness, the discomfort of moving around—and we accept it. Just as our social setting gradually conditions us to accept our decreased health, so the gradual descent of our personal health conditions us to accept it.

Scott puts it this way:

> Deception convinces us that there really aren't any chains, and that our so-called prison isn't all that bad a place ... Deceived, we start decorating our chains and develop designer syndromes to explain them away ... We accept our chains and resign ourselves to confinement in prison cells of disease. We lose hope and ... try to make ourselves at home and comfortable in our cell.[2]

In other words, we take drugs to mask the symptoms, dress to cover the weight, and do nothing to stop the slow decline—and usually surround ourselves with people who are doing the same thing. It's even more perilous if we surround ourselves with people who ridicule our attempts to get in shape, as we'll see in the next section.

The Spiritual Reason We Gain Weight

Billions of dollars have been spent trying to corner the market on diet and weight loss, but most solutions ignore the spiritual issue behind our struggle.

Here it is: The challenge we face plays directly into

our sin nature, which is naturally disposed toward comfort and ease and naturally inclined against sacrifice or denial of any kind. To make matters worse, losing one pound doesn't feel like it makes any difference at all, even though losing a pound can be difficult to do. The sacrifice-to-reward ratio is out of whack, particularly if you're struggling alongside a person who doesn't share your values.

Let's say you spend an entire week denying yourself bread and dessert. You watch your calories, work out on the StairMaster, and take a thirty-minute walk at least five or six days. Seven days later, you weigh yourself and discover that you've lost one pound.

Do your pants fit any better? Probably not. Do you notice any more energy? Unlikely. And yet the struggle was real. Think of all the time you spent exercising, all the sweets you denied yourself—and you lost just one pound?

Let's say you have a friend who is laughing at your efforts. The whole week, she has been eating her favorite comfort foods while you exercised, drinking sugary drinks while you sipped your water, consuming whatever she wanted off the menu. At the end of that week, she gained one pound.

Are her pants any tighter? No, they're not. Does she feel much heavier? Not likely. And yet she enjoyed the week so much more!

This is the spiritual struggle toward physical fitness: The initial sacrifice seems so great compared to the minuscule immediate benefits, while the negative consequences seem relatively minor compared to the instant enjoyment of overeating and ignoring exercise.

If you have a short-term view, you're going to give in. You need the spiritual strength and motivation to take it out a little further. If you continue in your sacrifice for ten weeks and lose ten pounds, and your friend continues in her excess and leisure for ten weeks and gains ten pounds, that's a twenty-pound swing. Now, your clothes *will* fit a bit better, and hers *will* be tighter, and both of you *will* notice a difference in energy level and overall health.

If you were overweight and I could miraculously remove fifty pounds from you for one hour, you would feel the difference and be highly motivated to do whatever it would take to make this be your normal state. But the problem is that we don't gain or lose weight that way. Losing one or two pounds doesn't feel much different to you on a day-to-day, week-to-week basis; gaining three pounds back is hardly noticeable. This phenomenon encourages slow weight *gain*, even as it discourages steady weight *loss*. Because the negative impact doesn't feel much worse and the positive impact doesn't feel much better, we're simply not motivated to get to the place where, long term, the difference can be tremendous.

That's why we need spiritual strength and biblical motivation to persevere through the temptation and stay the course. If our pursuit is simply therapeutic, we're facing almost impossible odds (unless we happen to be particularly vain). And that's also why it helps to have encouraging people around us who are on the same pursuit.

You Are My Inspiration

A true friend isn't always one who *accepts* us; sometimes a friend's job is to *inspire* us. Henry Van Dyke, a Princeton professor and clergyman, once said that the mark of a true friend is someone who makes you want to be at your best when you are with him.

Are you setting up a social base that inspires you to be the best man or woman you can be? Or is your group of friends and advisers giving up and giving in to the most common spiritual enemies of our age? Does your doctor address your symptoms, or does she address your decisions? Is your pastor strong enough to occasionally confront your disobedience?

We think the most loving thing we can do is to make someone feel good about themselves, no matter what, and the worst thing we can do is make them feel bad about themselves, but what if ignoring the truth is allowing or even encouraging a condition to continue that may take a decade or more off our friend's life? Is that *love* as the Bible defines it?

It's interesting that the church is more cautious of anorexia, which, all told, afflicts far fewer people, than it is of unchecked overeating, which captures millions. There's some sense in this: true anorexia is often a life-threatening condition, while obesity kills much more slowly. But anorexia is used almost as a joke when someone decides to get fit: "Well," she is warned, "don't get all anorexic on us." Why don't we ever say, "Don't get all gluttonous on us"?

Our priorities are almost comical. On the day I had run a marathon and was hobbling around at a group dinner, a concerned Christian woman pulled my wife aside and said, "I just don't think it's healthy for a man Gary's age to be running that far. It just *can't* be good for him."

Lisa had to bite her tongue, as this woman's husband is at least seventy-five pounds overweight and completely sedentary. Lisa wanted to know if this woman had ever said to *her* husband, "Hey, don't you think that eating too much and never exercising might not be healthy for you?"

The reality is that overeating and obesity kill far more people than anorexia or exercise. Yes, I know —every year a few people die running marathons.* I'm not suggesting that running marathons is healthy or even advisable. Training for 5K runs certainly is a healthy activity, but marathons may indeed be pushing it. I am certainly not advocating that Christians start viewing the completion of a marathon as an admirable life goal; for me, it is more obsession than spiritual discipline.

---

*Those who die under the age of thirty usually have an undiagnosed heart defect. Those marathoners who die over thirty years of age frequently failed to train extensively enough for such a long run (twenty-six miles is certainly not a distance to be trifled with).

Exercise certainly has its share of excesses that we need to guard against. Without denying these legitimate concerns, isn't it possible to recognize that ignoring excessive eating and laziness is affecting our witness, our health, and our personal lives? Simply ignoring this so that others don't feel momentary conviction can't be the best option.

It simply *can't*.

Let's be honest about the current level of Christian influence. Sociologist Kenneth Ferraro has found that religious practice in the United States correlates positively with obesity — *and Christians are the heaviest of all*.[3] An ordained friend of mine once joked that some Christian conferences could be written up as "50 souls saved, 500 bodies overfed."

Being silent about eating too much because we don't want to sound judgmental, or refusing to address laziness because it can sound elitist or we think it's none of our business, is to allow and even encourage fellow church members to live lives in which there is no inspiration to be made holy, useful to the Master, and prepared to do any good work. Let's create a new kind of environmental influence — one that demonstrates how we treat our bodies as a form of Christian stewardship, a vehicle for evangelism, and preparation for the good work that God has planned for us to do.

8

THE SILENT MURDERER

Laziness is the great spiritual assassin of our time. It kills our bodies; it kills our bank accounts. It kills marriages and parental relationships. It kills businesses and governments. It kills everything it touches.

It usually acts slowly, taking its time to carry out its venomous assault that often proves deadly.

Laziness is more than a sin — it's an attitude that undercuts our sense of duty to God and our obligation to our neighbor, and an attitude that wastes our lives. Julian of Norwich, a medieval anchorite, warns that "sloth and time wasting" are the "beginning of sin."[1] Brother Giles, an early Franciscan monk, advises that "the lazy man loses this world and the other, without doing any good to himself or others."[2]

Laziness is an attitude that puts one's personal comfort above all else — if I don't feel like it, why do it? If it's uncomfortable, why bother? If it's not fun, what's the use? Laziness ignores any sense of obligation and defines sin exclusively as something we shouldn't do (conveniently forgetting all that we *are* commanded to do), and it ends up wasting our lives in a spectacularly nonscandalous fashion so that we don't see just how destructive it is.

When we are neglectful with our physical bodies, part of us dies. We can avoid the wisdom of exercise and responsible eating, but we do so at our peril and accordingly will miss many opportunities to do good works. An out-of-shape Christian loses the will, inclination, and ability to enjoy much of life because physical activity becomes too taxing. He or she wants to sleep more, eat more, and lie around more rather than be truly engaged in life.

If we are lazy in parenting, we will have less of a relationship with our children. If we are lazy in marriage, we will grow distant from our spouses. If we are lazy in our business, our finances will gradually erode until we become charity cases instead of generous givers. If we are lazy in our faith, we will even drift from God. Neglect and laziness kill the best things in life.

This entire book is focused on becoming "holy, useful to the Master, and prepared to do any good work." Laziness is one of the greatest, if not *the* greatest, enemies of this pursuit. *Good* is never an adjective that a slothful person would put in front of *work*. Fourteenth-century hermit Richard Rolle argues that the rise from death to life is, at least in part, a rise "from laziness to exercise in the service of God."[3] A Christian fully alive is active in every sense of the word, as much as she or he is able to be so under the providence and care of God.

In one very real and intense sense, laziness undercuts the image of God in us. Johannes Tauler* makes precisely this point:

> The Heavenly Father, in His divine attribute of Fatherhood, is pure activity. Everything in Him is activity, for it is by the act of self-comprehension that He begets His beloved Son, and both in an ineffable embrace breathe forth the Holy Spirit ... Now since God has made His creatures in His likeness, activity is inherent in all of them ... Is it surprising, then, that man, that noble creature, fashioned in God's Image, should resemble Him in His activity?[4]

Ask yourself: What is the opposite of God's activity and generosity? Wouldn't it be doing nothing and giving nothing?

In other words, laziness and neglect!

The Bible is ruthless in condemning laziness and in warning against its consequences in various arenas of life:

---

*Johannes Tauler (fourteenth century), a Dominican monk, was a disciple of Meister Eckhart and a key voice of the influential German mystics. He spent most of his life in the Order of Preachers, and his writings had a significant impact on Martin Luther.

Go to the ant, you sluggard;
    consider its ways and be wise!…
A little sleep, a little slumber,
    a little folding of the hands to rest —
and poverty will come on you like a thief
    and scarcity like an armed man.

Proverbs 6:6, 10–11

The craving of a sluggard will be the death of him,
    because his hands refuse to work.

Proverbs 21:25

We want each of you to show this same diligence to the very end, so that what you hope for may be fully realized. We do not want you to become lazy, but to imitate those who through faith and patience inherit what has been promised.

Hebrews 6:11–12

The ancients tackled laziness (which they called "sloth") with the same earnestness that they tackled excessive eating. Lorenzo Scupoli, a sixteenth-century priest of the Theatine order, whose book *Spiritual Combat* was deemed so insightful that it was adopted by the Orthodox Church as well as the Roman Catholic Church, wrote of the "miserable bondage of sloth, which not only hinders all spiritual progress, but also delivers you into the hands of your enemies."[5]

Did you catch that? Scupoli argues that laziness constitutes "miserable bondage" and hinders *all* spiritual progress. If we don't address this failing, *everything else we do will be threatened*. Laziness is that serious.

Spiritual Laziness

Being a Christian is the highest joy imaginable for any human being. It is also, however, hard work. Listen to Paul's account:

> One thing I do: Forgetting what is behind and straining toward what is ahead, I press on toward the goal to win the prize for which God has called me heavenward in Christ Jesus.
> All of us, then, who are mature should take such a view of things.
>
> Philippians 3:13–15

Consider the phrase "all of us, then, who are mature should." Paul isn't showcasing his piety here or nominating himself for a Christian of the Year award; he's laying down a standard to which *every believer* should aspire. According to his inspired words, a mature Christian will *strain* toward what is ahead. Commentator Jac. Müller writes, "The verb used here is very descriptive, and calls to mind the attitude of a runner on the course, who with body bent forward, hand stretched to the fore, and eye fixed on the goal, strains forward with the utmost exertion in pursuit of his purpose."[6]

The great Puritan Jonathan Edwards was as blunt as a man could be about this: "We are nothing if we are not in earnest about our faith, and if our wills and inclinations are not intensely exercised. The religious life contains things too great for us to be lukewarm."[7] He takes it one step further when he adds, "If there is a fight to be fought, or a race to be won, then it must be done with utmost earnestness. Without this there is no way of traveling the narrow road that leads to life. Sloth is therefore as damning as open rebellion."[8]

I mention this because many will say getting in shape physically, changing the way they eat, making time for exercise, being disciplined to work out even when they don't feel like it, is too much effort. It sounds like works-righteousness. It might even lead to legalism. And since laziness and overeating don't seem like scandalous sins, we let them slowly but steadily steal our health away.

This concession fosters an attitude that will eventually erode our spiritual life as well. Laziness is like pride—we can't turn it on and off. It becomes a part of who we are. If we coddle laziness in one area of our lives, we'll succumb to it in other areas too. Sins are, by nature, self-reproducing. Selfish people are selfish in every way. How they drive, how they spend their money, how they talk, and even how they serve is marked by selfishness. In the same way, if we become lazy with our physical health, we are likely to become lazy with our spiritual health. The reverse is also true. Cultivating discipline in physical fitness can make us more apt to be disciplined in spiritual fitness.

Can we value work as Paul did? I love his comments in 2 Timothy 2:6, when he tells his young protégé to "reflect" on the fact that it's the "hardworking farmer" who gets the first share of the crops. This is such a brilliant metaphor that it's sad I've never heard a pastor preach on it. Much of a farmer's work—unlike, say, that of an athlete, solider, or politician—is done behind the scenes, without any glory, applause, or excitement. Ancient farming, particularly in the days before mechanized harvesting, was grueling work based largely on perseverance and consistent effort. That's the metaphor Paul uses to describe the hard, often anonymous work of a Christian as he or she pursues God and is used by God.

The renowned John Stott warns, "This notion that Christian service is hard work is so unpopular in some happy-go-lucky Christian circles today that I feel the need to underline it ... It may be healthy for us to see what strong exertion [Paul] believed to be necessary in Christian service."[9] Indeed, as Stott points out, Paul —*the* champion of salvation by grace through faith —gloried in the fact that "I worked harder than all of them," explicitly referencing his hard work in 1 Corinthians 15:10; 2 Corinthians 6:5; and Philippians 2:16. Paul always ties his labor to God's energy and provision but never in a way that God's provision puts Paul to sleep, and certainly not as an invitation to a life of neglect.

Physical fitness is like farming. Much of the work that produces it is unseen. No one is applauding or even recognizing our efforts. But the life it creates can be used by God to bless and serve many. The "planting" is grueling; the harvest can be great.

Just a few verses later in 2 Timothy, Paul tells Timothy, "Do your best to present yourself to God as one

approved, a *worker* who does not need to be ashamed
..." (2:15, emphasis added).

The reason spiritual neglect and apathy are so devastating is that the act of pursuing God makes life so
much sweeter. When I am seeking and growing in
God, my marriage and parenting, my eating and drinking, my laughing and playing and work, take on a holy
hue. The delight I have in God seeps into everything
I do, and if there is anything that blocks this delight, I
lose my taste for it.

But when my heart is spiritually lazy, when I am not
pursuing and delighting in God, then even the most
pleasurable acts can become points of stress and frustration. I lose the wonder of life; my alienation from
God colors everything with a depressingly gray hue.
Jesus' statement that whoever has will be given more,
and whoever does not have will lose even that (Matthew 13:12), becomes particularly true for those who
walk with or without spiritual delight.

Lorenzo Scupoli warns that "from the slothful,
God by little and little withdraws the graces He had
bestowed upon them, while to the diligent He gives
more abundant graces and permits them at last to enter
into His joy."[10]

Up or Down

The ancient writers of the Christian classics viewed
the spiritual life as either an upward progression or a
downward spiral. To them, there was no plateau. We

are either growing or dying. That's why they feared, hated, and shunned laziness. Listen to Scupoli again:

> This vice of sloth, with its secret poison, will gradually kill not only the early and tender roots that would ultimately have produced habits of virtue, but also habits of virtue that are already formed. It will, like the worm in the wood, insensibly eat away and destroy the very marrow of the spiritual life.[11]

Henry Drummond also tackled spiritual laziness. He believed an intentional, purposeful effort is essential to spiritual growth:

> What makes a man a good cricketer? Practice. What makes a man a good artist, a good sculptor, a good musician? Practice. What makes a man a good linguist, a good stenographer? Practice. What makes a man a good man? Practice. Nothing else. There is nothing capricious about religion. We do not get the soul in different ways, under different laws, from those in which we got the body and the mind. If a man does not exercise his arm he develops no biceps muscle; and if a man does not exercise his soul, he acquires no muscle in his soul, no strength of character, no vigor of moral fiber, nor beauty of spiritual growth. Love is not a thing of enthusiastic emotion. It is a rich, strong, manly, vigorous expression of the whole round Christian character — the Christ-like nature in its fullest development.[12]

Doesn't this make sense? Don't we know from every other endeavor in life that to do nothing is to watch things disintegrate? That a business has to be managed, a garden has to be weeded, a body has to be washed, a child has to be parented? Why should we think it any different when it comes to the health of our souls?

Confronting spiritual laziness doesn't mean ignoring physical life to tend to spiritual concerns, however; on the contrary, Drummond urges us to use physical life as a primary training ground for spiritual growth:

> Do not quarrel therefore with your lot in life. Do not complain of its never-ceasing cares, its petty environment, the vexations you have to stand, the small and sordid souls you have to live and work with. Above all, do not resent temptation; do not be perplexed because it seems to thicken round you more and more, and ceases neither for effort nor for agony nor prayer. That is the practice, which God appoints you; and it is having its work in making you patient, and humble, and generous, and unselfish, and kind, and courteous. Do not grudge the hand that is moulding the still too shapeless image within you. It is growing more beautiful though you see it not, and every touch of temptation may add to its perfection.[13]

When I'm not spiritually lazy, instead of resenting petty (or even not so petty) annoyances, I can consciously use them to "practice" godliness and cultivate a Christlike spirit. Being slowed down by an overly cautious driver; cleaning a floor only to have someone accidentally mess it up again; having a coworker make a mistake or call in sick—these are the moments Drummond urges believers to learn from, even to embrace. God is helping us "practice" our patience, our humility, our spiritual maturity. Learning to die to ourselves is never easy.

My friend Candice Watters told me she can have an amazing quiet time early in the morning, with "deep, spiritual thoughts," but the minute the kids get up, demanding things and bickering, "all that spiritual stuff dissipates." But this Drummond quote has helped her understand that both the quiet time *and* the family time are God's chosen methods for shaping her soul.

"No man can become a saint in his sleep," Drummond advises, "and to fulfill the condition required demands a certain amount of prayer and meditation and time, just as improvement in any direction, bodily or mental, requires preparation and care."[14]

Here's the difference: trying aspects of life will happen whether we use them or not. Spiritual laziness leads to resentment; spiritual diligence spawns insight and transformation *from the exact same events*. Let us become intentional to use personal slights, inconveniences, acts of gossip and slander, times of difficulty, and even sickness as opportunities to grow in patience and understanding and humility instead of bitterly resenting each one.

Living a life of diligent labor, faithfully discharging

all the duties God has given us, is the most fulfilling life any of us can ever live. It's the life we are designed to live. It's the life that on our deathbeds we will wish we had lived (or be grateful for those times we did live it). In the end, the *last* thing I want to hear from my Lord is, "You wicked, lazy servant!" (Matthew 25:26). Instead, don't we all long to hear, "Well done, good and faithful servant!" (verse 21)?

Let's cultivate hearts *and bodies* that will lead to this end.

LET'S GET PHYSICAL

Up to this point, we've been discussing fitness, excessive and indulgent eating, and laziness from a fairly high-minded perspective—how they affect our souls, what they do to our witness, the ways they impact our relationship with God. For one short chapter, let's get physical. Since we are called to be stewards of everything that God has given us, we need to be honest about the benefits and the damage of our health-related choices.

The Good News

Before we look at how devastating being out of shape can be to our overall health, let's look at the positive benefits of exercise and fitness.

According to Drs. Mehmet Oz and Michael Roizen,

"Your level of physical activity is the single most important predictor of whether you will look old and decrepit by age 62 or 102. Humans are designed to be physically active. The project of staying young is not about avoiding disease; it's about avoiding frailty."[1]

When we talk about becoming useful to God, I love this take: fitness isn't about avoiding disease; it's about avoiding frailty. I've noticed in my travels that there can be an astonishing difference between someone who is seventy years old and looks fifty-five and someone who is fifty-five and moves like someone who is seventy. Some of this is no doubt genetic, but lifestyle choices can make a significant impact. Dr. Steven Hawkins, a professor of exercise science, insists, "There's a big difference between biological age (how old your body says you are) and chronological age (how old the calendar says you are). The geological ages of runners are at least 10 years younger than their chronological ones, and the gap widens with time."[2] Within certain limits, we can greatly impact the quality of life that faces us in our senior years. According to Drs. Oz and Roizen, "Physical activity is underrated in terms of helping you stay vital and keep you from disintegrating."[3]

This is true *before* we become "elderly." In the busy years of my thirties, I allowed physical fitness to slide. I was working two jobs, trying to stay connected with my wife and involved in the lives of three small children. Slowly but surely, five extra pounds of weight became ten, and then fifteen, and then twenty. It wasn't until my early forties that I finally said, "This has to stop."

A young adult who had heard me preach when I was in my thirties came up to me after a talk I had given (I was now in my early forties) and said, "Gary, what happened? You look younger today than you did six years ago, and today you speak with twice the energy." The extra twenty pounds I carried affected me more than I realized.

In the short term, becoming fitter is about the quickest, easiest way to improve your overall quality of life, even if you don't actually lose weight. Tim Church, director of preventive medicine research at the Pennington Biomedical Research Center in Baton Rouge, Louisiana, found that women who did even ten minutes more exercise on a daily basis "felt more confident about doing everyday tasks—such as keeping up with their grandkids, climbing the stairs, and carrying in the groceries—and they felt better about themselves when they were in social situations." In this same study, "exercisers reported improvements in all areas of quality of life: agility, energy, overall health, mental health, emotional well-being, and functioning in social situations ... The more women exercised, the greater their improvements."[4]

Harvard Medical School psychiatry professor John Ratey, author of *Spark: The Revolutionary New Science of Exercise and the Brain*, has found that regular physical activity not only improves brain function but also helps to combat depression and anxiety.[5] According to Ratey, "A fast-paced workout boosts the production of a protein called brain-derived neurotrophic factor. I call it Miracle-Gro for the brain, and physical activity is one of the best ways to release this brain-nourishing protein."

This has so much anecdotal support that I'm not surprised by the scientific findings. If you've been sedentary and start to exercise, you're likely to feel miserable for a couple weeks, but once you can start working out without suffering every second of it, the mental benefits are enormous. The problem is, many people start out exercising for a week, feel only the suffering, and then give up before the mental benefits kick in.

Getting fit can be an arduous, even painful process; *living* fit is filled with much joy. When I'm in marathon shape and finish a long run without feeling spent, the boost I receive is enormous. I love God more. I love my wife and kids more. I'm dreaming of how I can serve God and be used by God. I'm more patient while driving. People may denounce physical exercise as "worldly," but I have found that it has enormous spiritual benefit.

And when it comes to fighting food indulgence, neurologically speaking, exercise is about the best possible substitute to overeating. Dr. David Kessler states, "A substantial body of science tells us that exercise engages the same neural regions [in our brains] as other mood-enhancing rewards and produces similar chemical responses."[6]

Let me put this plainly: researchers have discovered that you can get an emotional boost from an endorphin-producing workout, in which you lose weight, or a mental boost from eating a comfort food, in which you gain weight. The immediate mental reaction is the same, but one leads to health and vitality, while the other leads to disease and frailty.

It's not just about feeling good, though. Exercise also can improve the overall working of our brains, "preparing us to do any good work." According to Ratey, even a brisk walk can build better connections between brain cells and may increase the production of cells in the hippocampus, which is the region of the brain involved in learning and memory.

Ratey also cites exercise's ability to reduce stress and serve as a highly useful tool to fight back against smoking or alcohol addictions. He also believes it can benefit those with attention deficit disorder and even delay the onset of Alzheimer's. "We now have tons of studies that show regular physical activity can prevent the age-related brain fogginess that often develops by age 65."[7]

Finally, getting fit means you're also likely to die much more pleasantly. Dr. Cooper's clinic found that those who are fit tend to have a much more limited period of senility and diminished capacity. Such individuals tend to be highly functioning and relatively independent until they die rather suddenly. The "unfit" often live for years with limited capacity and slow deterioration, in a sense "crawling" toward death with greater misery and frustration. Of course, there is no guarantee — we've all known fit, healthy people who experience drawn-out, painful journeys toward death. But the evidence suggests that being fit can make this type of death much less common.

The Bad News

Now for the bad—even horrendous—news. Several studies released in 2009 reveal the stark consequences of obesity. Regardless of how one gets there, obesity can be devastating to a person's health. One study showed that obesity causes 100,500 new cases of cancer every year. The American Institute for Cancer Research discovered that excess body fat contributes to the following cancers: breast, endometrial, kidney, colorectal, pancreatic, esophageal, and gallbladder. Obesity also increases the risk for type 2 diabetes and heart disease.[8] A fairly recent Harvard study found that "obesity may soon surpass tobacco as the number one cause of cancer deaths."[9]

An extensive study of 900,000 people conducted by professors at Oxford University in England found that "adults who are obese—about 40 or more pounds over a healthy weight—may be cutting about three years off their lives, mostly from heart disease and stroke."[10] The news is even more grim for those who allow themselves to become 100 or more pounds over a healthy weight; they could be shortening their lives by as much as 10 years—an entire decade away from their children, grandchildren, and potential ministry.

I've been speaking about spiritual and physical

health, but Dr. Scott VanLue has found emotional applications as well. He warns that one of the most treacherous aspects of aging is that men lose testosterone just when their sons gain theirs.

> The worst case scenario is an alpha male with visceral fat. When testosterone converts to estrogen —which is what happens when muscle turns to fat—there's a natural predilection toward rage. So you have men with hormones that are more sensitive than ever [because of the estrogen], in the body of an alpha male that's set to explode. The overweight alpha male has more emotional sensitivity but less control, so he's easily set off. He is living with a son who is just growing into his own dose of testosterone. That's a natural setup for major conflict.[11]

Many pastors would treat a man's losing his temper and fighting with his son as a sin issue. While sin is clearly a factor, Scott treats it as a physiological one as well. The man will be much healthier, emotionally and relationally, if he loses some of the visceral fat that is converting his testosterone to estrogen at an unhealthy rate.

Not only are there physical and emotional consequences to weighing too much; there are financial ones as well. A study published in the journal *Obesity* found that obese twenty-somethings—those who are 30 or more pounds overweight—will have lifetime medical bills significantly above their normal-weight peers.[12]

Those 70 or more pounds overweight will incur even higher lifetime expenditures. A study conducted by George Washington University took into account things such as sick days, lost productivity, and the need for extra gasoline—and put the annual price tag of being obese at $4,879 for a woman and $2,646 for a man.[13]

These findings are all the more alarming when we consider the vast numbers of people who fall into the "overweight" categories. In fact, the statistics are downright staggering. About 66 percent of adults in the United States are either obese or overweight, with about one-third being obese.[14]

Yes, in one sense it costs time and money to get in shape. Staying unfit, however, brings its own costs and pains. The renowned Puritan Ralph Venning once wrote, "They who avoid suffering by sinning, sin themselves into worse suffering."[15] If I give in to every food desire, if I collapse in laziness every time I don't feel like exercising, I end up sinning myself into worse suffering than I would feel from hunger pangs or momentary exercise.

Let's be kind to our bodies, feeding them better foods and giving them sufficient exercise and occasionally denying them what they seem to demand. Let's become friends with our hearts, our lungs, our bellies, no longer asking them to bear the burden of temporary indulgence. Let's serve them so that they can serve us and help us live more meaningful and productive lives for God.

Fortified with Fitness

Nelson Mandela endured twenty-seven years of jail time on his way to living one of the most significant political lives of the twentieth century. By his own account, it was the lessons he learned in his youth as an amateur boxer and avid runner that gave him the strength to persevere.

Though his prison cell was not much bigger than a queen-sized bed (I've been in a replica of Mandela's cell that is set up in a South African museum—it was suffocating), Mandela dutifully ran in place and did push-ups and stomach crunches to keep himself from deteriorating. He was able to spend three of those twenty-seven years in a larger shared cell, which caused a bit of tension because he woke his cell mates up every morning at 5:00 a.m. with his one-hour runs around the cell's tight corners.[16]

Mandela didn't become president of South Africa until he was seventy-five years old. If he had let himself deteriorate physically during his incarceration, he may well not have been in any shape to lead after he was set free (certainly not to go strong until the age of eighty, which is how old he was when he left office). How many parents, grandparents, businesspeople, and pastors are cutting their careers short by making it impossible for their bodies and minds to continue well into their senior years?

God has given you many gifts and hard-won experience—are you maintaining your body in such a way that you can be a good steward of these gifts until God chooses to take you home? Are you a young person, in your teens or twenties, and forfeiting future productive years by falling into bad habits early in your life?

As a Christian, and as the father of two daughters and the husband of a wife, I applaud the church's desire and attempt to make all people feel welcomed, without judgment when it comes to body issues. The church should be a place of healing acceptance, affirmation, and encouragement. Within that ethic, however, can't we also find a way to value physical fitness, within its appropriate boundaries and priorities, since it is so clearly such a positive factor in mental, physical, and spiritual health? Indeed, shouldn't God's people —given our belief in God as the creator of our bodies, our acceptance of the call to be good stewards of everything God has given us, and the empowering presence of the Holy Spirit within us—be leading the charge in this contemporary battle?

Earlier ages did. Let's look at one such movement, which called itself "muscular Christianity."

MUSCULAR CHRISTIANITY

Famous psychologist G. Stanley Hall was perhaps a bit optimistic when he predicted that "among all the marvelous advances of Christianity ... in this land and century or any other lands and ages, the future historian of the church of Christ will place this movement of carrying the gospel to the body as one of the most epoch making."[1]

Hall was referring to "muscular Christianity," a late nineteenth-century movement birthed in England that stressed "manliness" and physical fitness as high Christian ideals. (Women, please don't be put off by the sexist language; the outdated verbiage contains great truth for every Christian, male and female.) This notion of "carrying the gospel to the body" was spawned in part by Englishmen who feared that the Anglican Church was becoming all too accepting of weak, out-of-shape bodies and effeminate men. It gained hold in the United States, in part because early Calvinism often considered "artificial exercise" an immoral waste of time, a sinful diversion, and thus indirectly fostered Christian leaders who claimed the mantle of spiritual leadership while carrying themselves in bodies that often spoke of ill health and physical laziness.

Among females, this neglect of the body led to numerous women being diagnosed as "neurasthenics," characterized by body aches, excessive worry, hypochondria, depression, digestive problems, persistent exhaustion, and inability to engage in life at any meaningful level. This was rife among women who could afford not to work, and the sad remedy was often a "rest cure," which never worked. These women needed to get their bodies in shape. Lying around the house waiting to get well was the source of their problem, not the solution.

Though undoubtedly deplorable sexism existed in this movement, astute women supporters picked up the truth behind muscular Christianity and challenged women as much as men. Fitness advocate Helen McKinstry asked what man contemplating marriage would choose a "delicate, anaemic, hothouse plant type of girl" over a "strong, full-blooded, physically courageous woman, a companion for her husband on the golf links and a playmate with her children?"[2]

Of course, even this sounds sexist to contemporary ears (getting in shape because otherwise men won't want you), but some, such as YWCA secretary Mary

Dunn, called women to fitness for the sake of the spiritual challenge that lay before them:

> Muscular women wanted, young women. What kind? Those to whom the Lord can say, "Do this or that for me," and who can respond to the hardest command, the carrying out of which will mean endurance, a knowledge of the principles of the conservation of energy and the putting forth of will power through bodily power. It will mean the clear shining of a flowing soul through a transparent medium, instead of the cloudy glass of an ... ill-used body.[3]

For Service

Muscular Christianity (MC) wasn't about bodybuilding for the sake of looking good, but rather about having a body that was fit for active service to God. Weak or out-of-shape men and locked-away neurasthenic women, supporters argued, not only live shorter and less effective lives, but they have less energy, command less respect, and provide less of a witness to the world. This is an ancient truth. The second-century bishop Irenaeus wrote, "The glory of God is man fully alive."

An early proponent of muscular Christianity, C. T. Studd, was one of the most accomplished cricket players of his day. While he eventually regretted having made cricket an idol, he remained grateful for the lessons that competing taught him—lessons such as the importance of self-denial, perseverance, courage, and the like. All these directly fed into a triumphant Christian life, suggesting that, for the redeemed, *thoughtfully* competing in sports can feed Christlikeness. In fact, James Naismith (a muscular Christianity proponent) invented the game of basketball as a means to evangelize people about morality and Christian values.[4]

These women and men understood — and we desperately need to recapture this today — that physical fitness can provide a fertile seedbed for spiritual growth *and* that physical laziness and an undisciplined attitude toward food can corrupt our souls. G. Stanley Hall argued that, sadly, many Christians were blind to the wonderful, life-enhancing aspects of "physical vigor," while also being ignorant to "how dangerously near weakness often is to wickedness."[5]

The Strenuous Life

To counteract soft, urban living, MC supporters coined the phrase "the strenuous life." Though some adherents unwisely discounted "book learning and study," others argued for the need for young people to work hard at their studies while also becoming physically fit, believing a whole person doesn't neglect any aspect of his or her being. Yale mathematics professor Eugene Richards warned that "the corruption of the body by sloth and effeminate luxury was followed by a mental decline, just as softness and weakness of mind ... have always gone hand in hand with ... enfeebled bodies."[6]

The thinking was that to live an influential, fruit-filled Christian life required a toughness, a hardy spirit, a confronting and facing of challenges, a learning to deal with failure without giving in to it, and a rising up to keep moving forward—each of these is a lesson that can be learned through sports. Actively fighting temptation, overcoming fears to step out in ministry, learning to work together as a team, handling defeat with grace and victory with humility, developing the courage to face an opponent who honestly (and perhaps quite rightly) scares you—these are characteristics of a woman or man who is being trained to engage in vigorous spiritual warfare.

Soft people who frequently complain about the smallest annoyances, who give in to laziness and excess, who expect others to work so that they can rest, who collapse into passive entertainment instead of active exercise—these are souls custom-made to become all but irrelevant in kingdom warfare. They are no threat to anyone—least of all to Satan.

MC supporters believed that the lack of teaching about the strenuous life was chasing the best and brightest youth from Christian churches. As one leader put it, "There is not enough of effort, of struggle in the typical church life of today to win young men in the church," for a "flowery bed of ease does not appeal to a fellow who has any manhood in him."[7]

By advocating sports, they weren't suggesting we needed to get competitive, but that physical fitness, on its own, has an enormous impact on our overall sense of well-being, and thus on our ministry and spiritual life as well. One clergyman wrote that taking up bike riding saved him from "monotony" and ill health: "[Along] came my bicycle, and, as if by magic, away went the spirits that had tormented me so long, and as their cloven feet and writhing tails disappeared in the dark past I was met by the laughing, beautiful faces of the spirits of health and cheerfulness."[8]

How many pastors or tired women executives could bring renewed vigor and joy into their lives simply by dusting off their bike seats, oiling up the chains, and making regular rides a part of their schedule? How many moms and dads could increase their energy levels substantially by going with their children to the pool and taking turns swimming laps while their kids play, instead of simply reading a book or newspaper as they sit on bleachers?

Chasing the Challenge

Nineteenth- and early twentieth-century leaders found that one of the great stumbling blocks to church growth in their day was that Christianity didn't offer much of a challenge. Salvation was offered free and unearned; church work consisted of committee meetings and teas; the main form of worship was singing flowery songs — not the stuff at all that would interest men and women who crave a challenge or who are struggling to build or run a business. One Baptist minister put it this way: "Men do not find enough to do in the church of that which requires skill and courage. There is too great a contrast between the strenuous business life to which they are accustomed and the lifeless committee work upon petty things to which they are invited."[9]

The same challenge exists today. Are our churches places where vibrant men and women embrace life with all its challenges and struggles and boldly move forward and inspire others, or are they places of committees, romantic songs, and disappointed people? We should be asking ourselves how we can become places of outreach that love, affirm, and build up the sick, the lonely, the recovering addicts, and the weak, while affirming the call to become strong, fit, and active servants.

Here is where the church has made a costly mistake. We take Paul's words to the Corinthians about God using the weak things of the world to shame the strong to be promoting *weakness* when in fact he is promoting *humility*. Listen carefully to what Paul says:

> Not many of you were wise by human standards; not many were influential; not many were of noble birth. But God chose the foolish things of the world to shame the wise; God chose the weak things of the world to shame the strong. He chose the lowly things of this world and the despised things — and the things that are not — to nullify the things that are, *so that no one may boast before him.*
>
> 1 Corinthians 1:26 – 29, emphasis added

A clear (but not the only) emphasis of this teaching

is that any of our boasting is to be boasting "in the Lord" (verse 31). As Gordon Fee explains, "Paul does not glory in his weaknesses for their own sake ... Rather, he does so to remind the Corinthians ... that the real power does not lie in the person or presentation ... but in the work of the Spirit."[10]

When Paul writes, "Brothers and sisters, think of what you were when you were called. Not many of you were wise by human standards ... But God chose the foolish things of the world to shame the wise" (verses 26–27), would any serious teacher suggest that academic study therefore doesn't matter, that we can remain ignorant, ill-informed, and uneducated, and glorify God in all of this? No! It means we study hard *in the fear of God*, embracing *his* wisdom and revelation, all the while adopting his humility.

In the same way, our physical weakness and laziness may be indicators of what we *were* when we were called, but becoming fully alive in Christ means we are invited to a new life, a full life, a vigorous and strenuous life of service.

The only alternative is to suggest that, somehow, to be ignorant, uneducated, and weak is the holiest state we can attain (and Christianity has had its extreme ascetics who believed and lived exactly this). Yet Paul himself suggests later in this letter that we should remember that we are not our own, that we were bought at a price, and therefore we should honor God with our bodies (6:19–20).

This doesn't mean our churches should be filled

with Olympic athletes. There are many church members for whom good health is not an option, who deal with multiple disabilities or illnesses. These dear saints can honor God with their bodies even more than those who are athletically gifted, by means of their spirit, perseverance, and brave acceptance of their limitations. *In no way* am I suggesting (nor do I believe) that only healthy, fit people honor God. Persevering in the face of disability takes more courage and perseverance than most of us will ever know.

Again, our emphasis is on silver souls, not outward appearance, and any strong soul is anchored by humility. Paul warns that knowledge, on its own, "puffs up" (1 Corinthians 8:1). The same can be true of physical fitness. Bodybuilding, marathon running, golfing, gymnastics—*any* sport can give way to selfish ambition and pride. But we would never suggest shunning knowledge and study because learning can lead to arrogance; why, then, would we suggest that we should shun physical fitness and achievement because they also might lead to sin?

It's the pride, not the ability or excellence, that dishonors God.

An early YMCA speaker believed that dropping this sense of the challenge of Christianity is what was keeping so many teenage and twenty-something men out of church (the same problem exists today). He argued that churches made religion "too easy and too cheap" and suggested that if they would "promise young men battles instead of feasts, swords instead of prizes, campaigns instead of comforts," the "heroic which lies deep in every man will leap in response."[11]

Student Volunteer Movement leader and muscular Christianity proponent John Mott (who turned down offers to become president of Princeton and a dean at Yale in order to focus on his evangelistic efforts with youth) energized and enlisted an entire generation of young men by stressing the challenges facing the world and the church, and how important it was for brave, fit, vibrantly alive, and strong people to step forward to confront these problems. It was MC's belief that a young man who doesn't see himself as part of the solution will inevitably become part of the problem. If the energy of young males isn't channeled to help others and build something positive, it will be abused to cause problems, wreak havoc, and unleash chaos. Idleness and softness lead to moral decline, just as vision and courage tend to foster moral character.

I've heard modern researchers lament the fact that 75 percent of our evangelical youth drop out of church, but in the early 1900s, the attrition rate for boys aged twelve to eighteen was similar, between 60 to 80 percent. Churches began to discover that trying to amuse boys or creating a "goody-goody, wishy-washy, ultra-feminine atmosphere" didn't appeal to young men, who needed to have their "soldier-like instincts" awakened on behalf of Christ's kingdom.[12] A high regard for "the strenuous life" could be a message that needs to be resurrected today.

Every historical Christian movement should be critiqued. They all have blind spots and unhealthy emphases and thus are often dismissed entirely because of these quibbles. But there is still much in MC we can embrace, beginning with the biblical call to become physically fit for spiritual purposes. Some of the MC proponent's attacks on study—pitting the mind against the body, for instance, rather than calling people to become fully alive in *all* aspects of being human— were unfortunate, as were some of the emphases of those in the "social gospel" camp, but let's keep our ears open to the challenging, historic, and biblical message of "taking the gospel to the body."

THE THREE-HUNDRED-POUND PASTOR:
CHANGING THE CHURCH CULTURE

Three hundred pounds.

Mark Bejsovec, a youth pastor, looked at the scale and couldn't believe what he was seeing. As a younger man, he had always been in pretty good shape, able to eat what he liked without worrying about gaining weight. During his high school football playing days, he carried just 186 pounds on his six-foot-two frame. He was the picture of health.

At twenty-six, his metabolism started to slow down; at thirty-two, it felt like it had stopped.

Soon, Mark was gaining about five pounds per month. At first, he rationalized it. "Well, I'm putting on some weight, but I'm still OK."

In fact, as an extrovert, Mark used his weight like a tool. It made him seem funnier. He could push out his stomach until he looked like he was eight months pregnant, and the kids in his ministry would laugh: "You look like you've got twins!" Making fun of himself invited the kids to make fun of him as well, and though Mark laughed on the outside, on the inside he began to grieve.

When he got home, he would look in the mirror and ask himself, "Man, what happened?"

In Mark's second year of full-time ministry, when he was in his midthirties, he began to sense God speaking to him about his physical condition.

"I looked into Scripture, specifically at the men in the Bible who assumed leadership roles, and wondered how they must have looked. I couldn't find anyone in leadership who was overweight."

Daniel 1:8 spoke most strongly to him. Here "Daniel resolved not to defile himself" by eating inappropriate food. Though this passage addresses food prohibited for religious reasons, a clear health element is involved, as Daniel and his friends emerge from their eating experiment looking healthier and fitter than anyone else.

"The fact that Daniel accepted the role God had called him to," said Mark, "even with his body, spoke dramatically into my life. Because Daniel was obedient, God turned around and honored him and gave him all understanding. I asked myself, How much am I missing out on because I have not been honoring God with my body?"

Another passage that challenged Mark was 2 Samuel 23:8–10, the story of David's mighty warriors. In particular there were Josheb-Basshebeth, who took out eight hundred men in one battle, and Eleazar, whose hand grew so sore from the fighting that it "froze to the sword." Mark said, "I can only imagine their physique and training; they were obviously in great shape and took care of their bodies, and God took care of them in battle and gave them great victory."

Reflecting on these passages convicted Mark of the need to look at his life from a broader perspective. "If I was addressing only spiritual issues but not the physical ones, I considered I would be less useful to the Lord in my ministry. If I was going to remain in ministry, I needed to honor God with all my heart, all my soul, all my mind, and also all my body."

Mark decided to quit his former eating habits cold turkey. "Overnight, I was done with sodas, sugar, cake, candy, cookies—all of them—and I lived that way for nine months." He also focused on filling himself with "good things," like nuts, vegetables, and good carbohydrates. There was no official diet, but rather greater sensitivity to what he was eating.

Because he had small children in his house, Mark found it particularly difficult to avoid the cake, ice cream, and cookies. "But what I found is that, just as with Daniel, the Lord gave me strength. God had begun to build in me a resistance until I came to the conclusion that my life is OK without this."

In the beginning there *were* occasional moments of hunger, but eventually his body seemed to reset itself. Within a month, he noticed that the portions of the meals he ate had shrunk, and the sickly bloated feeling had begun to go away, along with a few body bulges.

Just as happened with Karen (see her story in chapter 2), when his weight started coming off, Mark experienced a rush of positive energy. "I started feeling more affirmed, my self-esteem went up, and my relationship with God grew. It's not that my previous life didn't honor God, but now it felt like I was living like God designed me to live."

About nine months later, Mark had lost almost seventy pounds. He reached a point where he could occasionally have a piece of cake or a bowl of ice cream with his kids, but he never went back to abusing those as frequent indulgences.

Working with Weight

Mark's story — gradual weight gain in his late twenties and thirties until it snowballs out of control — is an increasingly common one in North America. As a youth pastor, Mark is keenly aware of how weight issues can hold young people back — particularly when the church is silent on this issue.

"We need to train young people to know that the way they are eating isn't sustainable. They may have faster metabolisms now, but if they aren't taught to eat better, once their metabolism slows, they'll face the same battle I did."

Mark points out that his parents never raised any issues about his eating, mainly because as an athlete he had stayed trim and fit. Who could blame them? Like most of us, they were focused on the *physical result*, not the *spiritual challenge*, of eating and fitness.

It wasn't just his parents who remained silent; the entire church joined in. Even after his weight reached three hundred pounds, not a single Christian approached Mark out of loving concern for his health, even though he admits, "If anyone had come to me in love, it would have been helpful."

He mirrors Karen's thoughts on this when he states, "We live in an acceptance-oriented society, where people are more afraid of hurting feelings than speaking the truth in love." Rather than challenge him about his weight, people actually tried to *encourage* him.

"You're looking great, Mark."

"Dude, I weigh three hundred pounds!"

"Well, you carry it well."

Mark never said what he thought. "Oh yeah? Want me to take off my shirt?"

God bless those people who wanted to encourage and accept a brother struggling with weight issues. There is much to commend in their concern. But isn't there also a place for raising issues of health and bodily stewardship, calling people out of harmful patterns of living?

Critiquing Our Own Church Culture

Evangelical Christians are famous for talking down popular culture, so why don't we, for once, challenge our *own* culture — our evangelical church culture? Has our obsession with appearing loving, tolerant, and accepting in contrast to the old fundamentalist methods of condemnation and legalism gotten out of balance?* I'm not suggesting we ever depart from a gospel of grace; I'm asking whether we may be neglecting the gospel of truth.

In the book of Malachi, God praises Levi because "he walked with me in peace and uprightness *and turned many from sin*" (2:6, emphasis added). In the same chapter, God condemns many in Israel because they "weary" him by saying "All who do evil are good in the eyes of the LORD, and he is pleased with them" (verse 17).

Even as we (commendably) want people to know they are loved, are we neglecting the truth that they also need to live in a spirit of repentance and openness to God's transforming work? Is it possible that telling people they are doing fine when they really aren't wearies God, as testified to in the book of Malachi?

I surely don't want to return to an overly pietistic, performance-oriented, shame-based legalism — who

---

*It certainly isn't fair or accurate to label all fundamentalists as judgmental, condemning, and legalistic. I'm speaking to the *perception* often expressed by our society and by other elements within the church.

does? But as God's representatives, we *are* called to urge others to turn from sin and to testify to God's will, however imperfectly we live it out ourselves, because a life of holiness is the most wonderful, meaningful, joy-filled, abundant life there is.

Romans 6:23 contrasts what life is like in obedience and disobedience. Paul states that the "wages of sin is death." The Greek word translated "wages" most accurately today would refer to minimum wage. It's a paltry, pathetic sum. Sin may grant a little pleasure, but its payment is relative to the person who cleans tables at the local mall's food court. On the other hand, "the gift of God is eternal life in Christ Jesus." The word for "gift" is more like "bonus." Not only does God pay a great salary, but he offers a bonus. His servants are like the Wall Street traders in December who get huge payouts on top of already abundant salaries.

When I leave someone in a life of disobedience because I don't want to risk offending him or risk having him think I'm not nice, I am essentially confining him to "minimum wage" existence — subsistence-level living. When he becomes a slave "to righteousness leading to holiness" (verse 19), he is elevated to bonus-supported living. How loving is it to allow someone to barely scrape by when God is offering truly abundant life?

All of this explains why I have told my wife that if I ever give into a sin and refuse to repent, I want her to go to another Christian brother, or even the church leadership, to plead her case. I don't want her to gossip about me or ridicule me or shame me, but if she deals with my rebellion redemptively, in love, in a biblical context, she's doing me a favor by continuing to confront my sin and refusing to let me be blinded by sin's deception. I know I have the capacity to make really stupid, even morally repugnant, decisions. I know sin makes me *increasingly* stupid. It can have a snowball effect. May God surround me with loving brothers and sisters who care enough to persist in calling me out of my stupidity so that I don't wreck my life with rebellion —because I know I am fully capable of doing so.

Much of our reluctance to call others out of their sin may be based on pride rather than love. We are sinfully people centered rather than God centered when we want people to feel accepted by us more than we want them to live in right standing before God. We have put ourselves in God's place, as if it is more important for *us and them* to be reconciled than for them to be in right standing with God. We are called to love everyone, but love doesn't mean making others feel comfortable, secure, and accepted by God in the midst of their rebellion.

Jesus loved the rich young ruler and the woman caught in adultery, but he called both of them to leave their lives of sin—the man his materialism, and the woman her adultery. When we redefine love to speak God's acceptance without also calling people to repentance, we risk judging Jesus himself, as if he were somehow deficient in his methods.

More Useful

When I ask Mark what has changed most about his life since he lost seventy pounds, he immediately responds, "Peace." As I've been saying all along, the physical change in his body has produced significant spiritual benefits.

He also believes it has made him, to use our language, more "useful to the Master and prepared to do any good work." Mark observes, "Let's be honest: there were times I was discredited because of the way I looked. When I talked to kids about self-control in other areas, they could look at me and understandably ask why I wasn't addressing *my* issues with food. But now, when I share my story, there's an added inspirational element. If I can do it, anyone can do it, and my weight loss has become an effective tool in my ministry."

Churches Fighting Back

One of the things Mark is now more sensitive about is how Christians routinely gather around food. Previous generations of Christians are famous for their beloved "church potlucks." It seems that just about every Sunday school class provides snacks, and younger Christians often meet at coffee shops, with calorie-laden drinks spicing up the conversation. Even at small group gatherings, it's assumed that someone is bringing something to eat.

I'm not suggesting that celebrating mealtimes is inappropriate—there is certainly a biblical place for these festivities. But if we value health and if we desire to honor God with our bodies, we can learn to exercise together as well as eat together.

I talked with some enthusiastic church members in the Midwest who organize a weekly workout group. They gather on Saturday mornings and then pray and go for walks or runs of various lengths. Because so many people take part, virtually every person can find a group to join. Volunteers set up aid stations along the route for those who run longer distances.

Here's what is brilliant about this plan: not only does it foster fellowship focused on getting in shape; it provides a wonderful opportunity for non-Christians to get to know Christians in a supportive, nonreligious context. If you've run or walked as part of a group for several months, it's a much more natural invitation when someone in the group says, "Hey, what are you doing for Easter? Have you thought of joining us *inside* tomorrow morning?"

Churches can organize bicycle rides, moms-pushing-strollers walks (or runs), adult soccer leagues, volleyball teams—you name it. If you have a Pilates class and get women to come inside the church building to attend, you've just removed one of the biggest stumbling blocks for visitors—the fear of entering a strange place.

Please don't misunderstand. Making delicious meals is a wonderful way to serve and love others. There's nothing wrong with communal meals and tasty snacks.

There *is* something wrong, however, about enabling someone who is trapped in an unhealthy pattern of living. If I give a couple I know well an expensive bottle of wine for their anniversary, that's generosity; if I knowingly give a bottle of wine to a recovering alcoholic, that's just flat-out mean.

Let's create room in our churches for conversations rooted in love as we show concern not just for a person's *emotional* well-being but for the *physical* well-being of that person too. Let's be more concerned about someone walking in right relationship with God than with whether that person thinks we are loving, accepting, and tolerant.

It takes just a little creativity for churches to make room for physical fitness, and when they do, they will fortify their members to become, like Mark, more useful to the Master and more prepared to do any good work.

STRONGER SHOULDERS

Kristin Armstrong had, in her words, "kind of floated" in her faith through her early adulthood. "It embarrasses me deeply to admit that there was a time in my life when I had no room for God. I was filled with ego, busyness, material things, and bubbles of emptiness."[1]

When she married a famous man (Lance Armstrong, seven-time winner of the Tour de France) and later went through an equally famous divorce, her faith reawakened.

"When you have that view of yourself as being self-reliant, and then everything starts to fall apart, and you respond by trying to work harder and you keep pushing harder until you realize you can't do it and you come up empty ... It's devastating and humbling. It felt like everything was falling out beneath me."

How does a mother of three tell her young children

that their home is about to be shattered? How does a woman relate to a man who used to be her best friend but who at times (but not now) felt more like an adversary? How does a woman who wanted nothing more than to share her entire life with a man begin to decide who gets what?

In Kristin's case, how does she forget her pain when she shops for groceries and sees her name and face splashed all over the pages of tabloid magazines lining the checkout stands?

The pain, the frustration, and the darkness of divorce have ripped the psyches of men and women for almost as long as marriage has existed. But this particular collapsing marriage created a new soul, a new home, and a renewed faith. God used physical and spiritual training to put a new Kristin back together.

Falling Apart

Already slim when she returned from Europe in August 2003, Kristin began looking alarmingly skinny as her marriage wound down. Two close friends, Paige and KT, noticed that Kristin wasn't eating much and was sleeping even less. She seemed racked by anxiety, was uncharacteristically sloppy, and was even a little scattered.

"Normally I'm a pretty sharp, together person," Kristin confides, and no one looking at her now would disagree. But divorce takes its toll. The personal pain of a dying romance can be paralyzing enough; add parental guilt, the burden of bearing others' judgment and condemnation, the endless practical details — lawyers, custody discussions, dividing the goods — in the end, no one survives divorce unscathed.

Yet the woman sitting across from me looks the very picture of health on her way to a workout (which she was). In that trying year of 2003, however, Kristin looked "haggard. I was a terrified woman. I was weak and wimpy and discouraged. I cried in the shower, at church, and anytime I drove alone."

One day Kristin was standing in her kitchen, frosting cupcakes for her son's class. "I was trying so hard to be normal, to go on smoothly with the regular duties of life. But suddenly it all seemed too much for me. I sat down and cried, still holding my frosting-covered spatula, shaking and broken."

With God-ordained timing, Paige let herself into the house, literally picked Kristin up off the floor, and helped her finish the frosting.

With the hard but kind words only friends can offer, Paige and KT eventually told Kristin, "You have three children to take care of. You can't afford to fall apart. You need some help. You need to get in shape" — but the help they offered wasn't just a consoling chat over a cup of coffee or piece of pie. It wasn't a simple Bible verse or a quick prayer that Kristin needed. More than a "spiritual vitamin" she needed a stronger soul.

So Paige and KT suggested Kristin train with them to run the Dallas White Rock Marathon.

Kristin had gone on short jogs before, mostly to lose

the "baby weight" following her pregnancies, but she had never even considered completing a marathon. Besides, couldn't this be considered cruel? What kind of friends would look at a tired woman who wasn't sleeping, who was losing weight she couldn't afford to lose, and who had suddenly been thrust into the harried world of a single parent and a public divorce, with all the increased responsibilities of doing alone what she used to do as a couple, and suggest that she add *running a marathon* to her to-do list?

In Kristin's words, "They knew I needed to gain the confidence of knowing I could work through pain on a physical level so that I could face the work ahead of me on emotional and spiritual levels."

Kristin's friends had tapped into the truth we've explored here: getting physically fit can help us face spiritual and relational challenges. It won't make those challenges go away, but it can give us stronger shoulders to face them.

The healing effects of Kristin's new training regimen soon became apparent. "For me, running was a catalyst for healing on all levels." Buoyed by food and improved sleep, along with the intense emotional bonding that comes from sweating through, suffering from, and talking on long runs, Kristin felt her strength and confidence return. Prior to a particularly brutal mediation session, Kristin spent the morning on a twenty-mile run. The endorphins and "good" weariness put her in a calm state of mind so that in the midst of what could have been an acrimonious encounter, Kristin calmly participated and said to herself, "I just ran twenty miles; *I can do this.*"

Kristin completed the Dallas White Rock Marathon four days before her divorce became final. As one part of her life—her marriage—was dying, another part of her life was being reborn. Spiritually and physically, in an intertwined reality, Kristin was literally becoming a new person, a new mom, a new friend, a new kind of Christian. She had run her way to a stronger, more mature soul.

Sinewy Endurance

As a person of faith, Kristin aspires to two character-istics in particular. The first is endurance. "Endurance is built through experience, repeatedly practicing the effort so that you have what it takes to reach comple-tion. Endurance is the confidence that you can with-stand pain."

Life is tough, so we must become tougher. If there's one thing that teaches you that you can withstand pain, it's training for a marathon. "When I ran at first, everything would hurt. I felt the fatigue in my legs, in my lungs, in just about every part of my body, but I gradually found that I could endure for longer bouts of time, and that carries over into every part of my life. I'm not just training for some race or event. For me, this is an ongoing part of my life, about who I'm becoming.

"Becoming fit means that, if you lose your job, your spouse walks out, or you discover you have a lump in your breast, you're strong and you have the endurance you need because life is going to get really tough. You need to be strong and you need to have endurance. Getting fit is *not* about what I look like in a pair of jeans; instead, I really care about being strong and having endurance spiritually."

Kristin believes that a Christian who has learned how to endure is a Christian who isn't as vulnerable to everyday challenges. One woman can face a dozen problems at once and display amazing peace, while another may have complete health, every luxury, and an abundant bank account and still be traumatized by fear and anxiety or relatively trivial challenges. The spiritual disciplines are the place to start, but their effectiveness is magnified when joined with physical discipline.

The enduring life is a solid life built over time — and physical training feeds into this. "As we run, we train our bodies, minds, and spirits, and our fitness levels in each category rise accordingly."

A single mom knows the need for endurance. The challenge of raising three kids on your own means that, when you have custody, everything is on your shoulders. You can't get tired and just take the day off. And the load doesn't lighten. It's day after day after day.

The second word Kristin uses to describe maturity (in addition to *endurance*) is *sinewy*. "I want to be a sinewy Christian, without a lot of fluff."

What does it mean to be a sinewy Christian? "A

sinewy Christian is lean, muscular, disciplined—not weak, flabby, indulgent.

"Go into any church. When you look at Jesus on the cross, he's sinewy. There's no fluff on him. That's not an analysis of him and his body, but his person. He was focused and intent. For us, it has to do with how we conduct ourselves, how we treat people. Physically, do you eat a lot of junk, have a lot of flab on you in general? I want to be lean; that has a lot to do with acquisitions, with food, just acquiring junk. I think of sinewy as being clean and lean."

She points out that many Christians become spiritually and physically flabby—complacent and lazy about life. "As Christians we're supposed to be growing and maturing. We're not supposed to get stagnant or lukewarm in our faith. 'Good enough' is often a far cry from 'best.' God calls us out of complacency. He wants us to be sharp and prepared. He wants to draw us further into contentment by challenging us to become the people he intended us to be."

Faith-Based Fitness

So what makes Kristin's attitude toward exercise different from the attitude of those who confess that they are unhealthily addicted to exercise or who live primarily for the physical and never give thought to the spiritual?

A reporter once asked Kristin's friend Paige about that, particularly as it related to Kristin. Could she be using running as an escape?

Paige responded, "Kristin's not running away *from* anything; she's running *to* something."

Kristin explains what Paige meant: "People running away from something, using running as an escape to avoid problems—there is something wrong there. That's more fear-based than faith-based fitness."

What marks her struggle as faith based? Kristin points out that our bodies aren't just flesh, blood, water, and organs; they are the dwelling place of the Holy Spirit. "Therefore honor God with your bodies" (1 Corinthians 6:20). She points out that "with so much emotional and spiritual revival going on during this time, we must not neglect our bodies. Our physical selves must be in balance with the progress made in other areas of our being. This means treating ourselves as holy dwelling places, as sanctuaries."

While this won't lead everyone (or even most people) to run marathons, the principle is still the same. "We can all take stock and find areas needing attention and improvement. We can better nourish and hydrate our bodies. We can get proper rest. We can improve our fitness. We can be mindful about our indulgences. We can choose to honor the Lord with the gift of sexuality by making godly choices."

Each day provides "a multitude of ways to improve the way we shelter the Holy Spirit of God."

Faith-based running is built up over time. You don't graduate from racing 5Ks to running a marathon in a week or even a month. Your body has to be built up and strengthened. Faith is the same way. There's no quick fix to spiritual maturity, no microwaved saints. God's women and men are cooked slowly, in a Crock-Pot, and allowed to stew.

Kristin isn't a fan of suffering for its own sake, but she appreciates what enduring suffering can accomplish: "There is no point to suffering if no redeeming good results from it. You are not being tested merely to receive a grade on your report card. You are being honed to become a blessing and an encouragement to others." In the language I've been using, we are being honed to "become useful to the Master and prepared to do any good work."

A New Life

So has it worked? Has this combination of physical and spiritual fitness created the life that Kristin believes God has called her to live?

Kristin says the divorce initially led her to feel "like a woman after a house fire, sifting through burned treasures in the ashes," but physical training helped her lift her eyes long enough to see that "sometimes it takes a pile of rubble to prepare the way for a major remodel."

After God began putting Kristin's life back together and as she grew stronger and godlier and more in love with her Creator, she began hearing comments like, "Something's different. Did you cut your hair?"

"No."

"Lose weight?"

"No." (Actually she had gained a bit—though it was muscle.)

"Have some 'work' done?"

"Absolutely not!"

"Huh. Well, *something* is different; I just can't put a finger on it."

Kristin testifies, "There is no transformation more deep or mysterious than when the Holy Spirit takes up residence within and begins to shine through. You are softer and lovelier than ever, yet you have never been stronger or more certain and direct. You are becoming an amalgamation of all the facets of woman that God intended when he created Eve."

Allow me to quote from Kristin's book, *Happily Ever After*, written to help women recover from the trauma of divorce. In one entry, Kristin writes:

> If I knew tomorrow was the last day of my life, I would get up early. I would make coffee and have my prayer time before the kids woke up. I would praise God for all the days He gave me. I would snuggle my children and make pancakes for breakfast in the midst of noise and chaos in my kitchen. I would pack lunches, braid hair, find shoes, brush teeth, and hand out backpacks. I'd probably drive to school in my pajamas. I'd pray a blessing over my children in the car and kiss everyone. After I was alone, I'd go running. I'd feel my lungs and legs burn and notice the way the sunlight filters through the trees along Town Lake. I would try to

meet a girlfriend for coffee. I would call my parents and my brother to say, 'Hi, how are you? I love you.'

In other words, on my final day, I would do the same exact things I do every day. I would live the life I am living right now. If I had to choose, I'd choose what I have.[2]

Are you facing a soul-shattering life change—a relational failure, a vocational challenge, a health crisis? Have you considered that getting physically fitter—not as a way of escape, but as a way of preparation—can give you stronger shoulders to face the battle ahead?

13

PURELY PRACTICAL

Now that I've laid out the spiritual principles behind a life of physical fitness — principles for becoming tougher internally and rejecting indulgence and laziness — let me offer some practical advice on how to apply all this.

What Is Fitness?

I don't pretend to be an expert in this area. From reading widely, however, I believe that Dr. Kenneth Cooper, in his book *Faith-Based Fitness*, gives the most precise summary of the findings of the majority of studies about generally healthy physical fitness:

- It's important to engage in regular, moderate endurance exercise.

- It's important to pursue a strength and flexibility training program throughout your life — and especially if you are middle-aged or older.

- It's important to emphasize low-fat, high-fiber foods in your diet.[1]

For me, fitness also requires watching my *quantity* of food. I simply feel better, spiritually and physically, when I eat less. Occasionally going to bed a little hungry does many good things for my soul, if not my body. And feeling lighter is worth far more than the momentary rush I get from overeating.

Fitness becomes even more important as we age. Dr. Cooper, speaking to women, puts it this way: "Physical protection against cardiovascular diseases is an act of *God* for women under fifty, but an act of *woman* for women over fifty."[2] What he means is that, prior to menopause, a woman's body seems to naturally fight much of the causes of early cardiovascular disease, but after menopause, when estrogen levels plummet, a woman "must pay closer attention to diet, exercise, and other preventive strategies to ward off heart disease and other threats to health."[3]

There are so many ways to become more physically active today that motivation is 99 percent of the battle. Many may say, "I don't have time," but what about the example of Dr. Emerson Eggerichs, bestselling author of *Love and Respect*? He has rigged up a "desk" that sits over a treadmill (I'm not making this up). In the course of walking while he works, Dr. Eggerichs puts in about twelve to thirteen miles a day without taking away a single minute from his work schedule. He checked with an exercise physiologist to make sure this walking was actually giving him the cardiovascular workout required to maintain health, and the specialist assured him it was.

If you have babies, there are strollers to use as you walk. If you prefer organized sports, just about every sizable city has soccer teams, volleyball leagues, or pickup basketball games to join. There has never been a generation for whom nonvocational exercise has been easier, more accessible, and in many ways, more enjoyable.

Getting in the Groove

Karen Yates, the mother of three whom we read about earlier, noticed how her babies could get into certain routines. "Feed them in the middle of the night, and the next night they would want the same thing. Do it a third night, and it was all over. The routine was set."

We adults are like this too. If I slip up and start eating too much on a sustained basis, I know I'm going to have to let my body get hungry until it resets and fits back into the old routine. I'll need to cut back the quantity, and at first, my stomach will scream out its defiance. But if I don't listen to it—if I break out of the routine of overeating—eventually my stomach will leave me be.

Earlier, I mentioned my habit of spot fasting in the evening. Once I'm in shape, I'll let myself break out occasionally on certain weekends, particularly Friday and Saturday evenings. But here's the thing: if I add Sunday evening to the break, I know there's going to be a battle on Monday. Three nights in a row, and my body is thinking, "Where's my snack?"

Since consistent overeating is what generally leads to weight gain, we need to fight against those patterns that regularly and thoughtlessly add more calories to our diets than we need. If you're used to consuming soft drinks with your lunch, it'll feel like a challenge to order ice water instead. Three weeks later, you won't even have to think about it. It's that initial breaking out of the pattern that takes the most effort—unless, like me, you let yourself slip up on vacation and have to go "off the wagon" all over again.

Breaking *any* pattern feels uncomfortable. This is why most of us will need to develop a new relationship with hunger pangs and daily exercise.

Get in a Group

For whatever reason, many women I talk to emphasize the relational component of exercise more than most men. Kristin Armstrong said that one of her favorite things about training for a marathon was reconnecting with friends on a regular basis. Karen Yates appreciated the opportunity to go to a gym and play volleyball, where the topic of conversation wasn't primarily about kid issues.

It's easier to blow off an exercise time if you're on your own. If you've already agreed to meet someone, you'll be more inclined to keep your appointment. So, women in particular, find some exercise partners. Add a social element into your fitness routines. Give a friend you want to get to know better a copy of this book and say, "Hey, let's take this seriously. When can we start?" Working out with a friend will help take your mind off the effort and is likely to make you more disciplined and increase the enjoyment of the entire experience. And the more you enjoy something, the more likely you are to stick with it.

Keep It Going

This teaching about the need to get or stay fit should not be reserved only for the megachurches that primarily serve those in their twenties, thirties, and forties. It is even more important for congregations that have people in their fifties, sixties, and beyond.

Professor Jeremy Morris from Liverpool, England, is known as the scientist who invented the field of physical activity epidemiology and health. Morris made the following observations at the age of ninety-four:

> So many bodily functions improve with exercise. The important thing is to carry it on into old age. My main concern now is physical activity in

old age. There's such scope there. There's such potential there.

It's very elementary physiology. We start losing muscle and losing cardiorespiratory, heart, and lung capability from our forties. Everybody does. Everybody. It's part of aging. Of course, if you're very fit, you start at a higher level, but the average person loses muscle at the rate of about 1 percent a year. And if you don't try to compensate for that —as you can to quite a large extent by exercise— by the time you get to be an old lady in the eighties, you may have lost half your muscle mass. And there's the basis for a lot of the frailty of old age."[4]

Modern lifestyles in the United States and many other countries now demand that we become proactive about adding exercise into our daily schedules, because otherwise we become all too sedentary. Morris again:

> We are the first generations in history, in the history of mankind, that have deliberately got to take exercise for health. You see, there used to be a lot of activity in occupation in your work and in getting about. In transport. And in the home. And this has gone down so drastically that we've all got to think in terms of deliberately taking exercise.[5]

A farmer who bales hay, a mail delivery person who walks her route, and a UPS man who delivers packages don't need to add exercise to their occupations. But those of us who work at desks can't afford not to use our leisure to do what used to be accomplished during the workday.

How Much Is Enough?

One of the most common "religious" arguments against physical fitness has to do with stewardship of time. I wrestle with this as much as anyone. Having so much to do, can I justify taking ninety minutes a day to ride a bike, play a game of racquetball, or swim laps — and then still have to take a shower?

The reality is, however, that exercise usually *adds* to our lives. A Harvard alumni study, which has tracked deaths among 17,000 men for more than two decades, suggests that "overall, each hour spent exercising adds about two hours to a person's life expectancy."[6]

Besides, it's a fallacy to suggest that exercise is comprised of "dead" hours. Many women find that going for a daily run or walk or participating in twice-weekly soccer or volleyball games is their best chance to connect with friends. I find my exercise time to be perfect for occasionally de-stressing, listening to a sermon, or thinking through a point for an upcoming talk or book. Many times, I just pray. This may be more difficult if my exercise was grudgingly carried out on an elliptical exercise machine at a health club, but this is only more reason to find a form of life-giving exercise that builds your soul while it strengthens your body.

I say all this before I depress you with the United

States Department of Agriculture's findings that now recommend exercise of between sixty and ninety minutes a day for people who mean to sustain weight loss. For cardiovascular health, we can get by on much less, but unless we're highly disciplined about what we put into our mouths, we need about this much time on our feet to actually *lose* weight or even maintain weight loss.

Some of you are going to start working out twenty minutes a day, four days a week, and give up when "nothing happens." This is not a fair test. It's a good start, but it won't serve the cause of actually losing weight, unless it is combined with disciplined eating. When a young college student goes out for a thirty-minute run and rewards herself with four Oreo cookies, the whole experience is actually a net calorie *gain*.

But please don't measure success primarily by weight loss. Remember, we're focusing on becoming stronger spiritually. Notice how much more patient you may be, or perhaps you're experiencing increased joy, zest, and energy for life. These are significant gains, regardless of the number on the bathroom scale.

The good news is that fitness actually matters more than body shape. Dr. Stephen Blair, of the University of South Carolina's Arnold School of Public Health, who previously worked at the Cooper Institute, states, "In our research, people who are obese but fit, according to cardiovascular measurement, actually have death rates half of normal-weight people who are unfit."[7]

Let Gentleness Be Your Friend

Some of you may be duly convicted that you need to address previous inattention to physical fitness, so you decide you're going to fix it *now*. May I suggest a bit of caution? A clear biblical principle is that what matters most is not so much where you've been as where you're headed. When getting in shape, overaggressiveness may be the pathway to defeat. Learn to take gentle steps.

The vast majority of us will give up if we try to overcome years of soft living with minutes of hard exercise. Once again, developing a silver soul is a *process*. If you're out of shape, walking a mile around a track while you pray could be a full workout for you — and nothing to be ashamed of. You're moving toward fitness, and that's what counts. No, you're not burning many calories at that rate. You'll never drop pounds or lose inches off your waistline with such limited physical exertion. *But you're on the path to greater spiritual and physical health.*

Find something you can enjoy — riding a bike, swimming, taking a walk, doing some cross-country skiing, working out on a rowing machine — or at least find a way to make a physical activity enjoyable. Listen to a sermon or music on your iPod. Do an activity with a friend or spouse. Watch a movie while you're on the treadmill.

If you hate something, you're not going to be able to pray while you're doing it. And if you're really sore, your spiritual thoughts will be eclipsed by the physical pain. I'm inviting you into a new way of life that is designed to reduce stress and make you more spiritually alive to God. Creating more stress and condemnation through embarking on overly ambitious programs will work against those aims.

From a physical perspective, Dr. George Blackburn, associate director of Harvard Medical School's Division of Nutrition, recommends the "10 percent rule": when you're trying to lose weight, lose no more than 10 percent over a period of three to six months, then hold that level for another six months before proceeding further. Dr. Blackburn believes this gives your body a chance to adjust to a lower "set point" (or typical body weight).[8] Because our bodies have complex systems designed to actually "defend" our current weight, trying to lose too much too quickly can become discouraging and ineffective.

From a spiritual perspective, I can't overstate the importance of embracing grace when addressing these issues. After we are convicted to address a long neglect, what matters most each day is not the body we have from our past, but what we're doing with our bodies in the present. This is what is pleasing to God: Am I being obedient *today* — right now?

This means I can worship and glorify God with a fat body or a fit body, with a muscular body or a skinny body, with an elderly body or a young body, with a disabled body or an athletic body. Because of grace, each day becomes an opportunity to worship and serve God with my body, regardless of what condition my past choices have left me in.

In the end, the gentle hand will be the winning hand. The soul that embraces God's grace and acceptance will be the victorious soul. Getting fit isn't about earning God's love but about being set free by God's love.

Give yourself time and enjoy the journey.

MEET MY FRIEND MORTY:
OUR ONGOING BATTLE AGAINST SIN

> But you, man of God, flee from all this, and pursue righteousness, godliness, faith, love, endurance and gentleness.
>
> 1 Timothy 6:11

Have you ever wanted something *really badly* but weren't sure you'd ever be able to get it? I'm sure most of your pursuits have been much nobler than mine, but from the time I was a boy, I dreamed of running in the Boston Marathon. It's the only marathon in the country that has qualification times, so it's not simply a matter of paying your money or setting aside a weekend. You have to run a fast enough qualifying time to get there.

My first marathon was all about finishing. During my second and third marathons, I gave qualifying for Boston everything I had but fell short.

I decided to increase my training mileage to make another serious attempt, but it led to plantar fasciitis, an excruciating heel condition that can take months to heal. The injury created a two-year gap between my third and fourth marathons.

When my doctor gave me clearance to run again, I had been sedentary for so long that when I laced up my shoes, even an 8:30 mile felt fast, and I thought to myself, "How will I ever run twenty-six miles at a much faster pace than this?"

When it comes to Boston, though, aging has it benefits. It gives you a whopping ten extra minutes to qualify when you turn forty-five years old. When I hit that chronological milestone, I knew all I had to do was finish a marathon in three hours and thirty minutes. I had already done that. Piece of cake, right?

I put in all the necessary miles and workouts and chose an ideal course — Grandma's Marathon in Duluth, Minnesota. It's a fast, scenic course, and I was ready to go. Because I had to travel by plane and stay in a hotel, though, the trip cost about a thousand dollars. This investment was sounding extreme to me, but Lisa was growing weary of living with an obsessed husband, so she even urged me on.

"Go get Boston," she told me.

When I woke up on marathon day, it turned out

to be a "black balloon day"—a heat/humidity caution alerting runners with health issues *not* to run, and others to adjust their pace accordingly. My body was ready to go, and the early miles clicked off ridiculously easy, but as the heat and humidity continued to climb, so did my mile times.

It ended up being my slowest marathon by almost a half hour. I was even pulled into the medical tent at the finish line to get rehydrated. As I lay on the cot getting a saline solution dropped into my veins, all I could think about was all those runs, those months of training, the agony of getting over plantar fasciitis, *one thousand dollars*—and Boston was farther away than ever ...

Back in my hotel room, more physically spent than I had ever been and thankful that I was still so dehydrated I didn't need to use the bathroom because I didn't have the energy to walk that far, my wife commiserated with me on the phone and finally suggested, "You know honey, maybe you're just not cut out to run fast enough. I mean, you said yourself that only 10 percent of those who run a marathon will ever qualify for Boston."

I didn't want to hear that. I didn't want to admit defeat, though I suspected she might be right.

I kept running but waited a year to make another earnest attempt. Lisa drove with me to Coeur d'Alene, Idaho (this time I wasn't willing to spend the money to fly somewhere). I ran a little more conservatively than

I did in Duluth, but not by much. The tough point, I knew, would come at mile 15. That's the crest of the one major hill on the course (which you run up twice). If I had something left in the gas tank after that, I figured I could get more aggressive.

I crested the hill at a 7:57 pace, thinking, *I didn't even lose time on the climb! Is there anything left?*

It's a glorious feeling to dig down in the tank at fifteen miles in a marathon and find a *lot* left. The next eight miles clicked by, but then, with just three miles left, when I was so close to qualifying it hurt to even think about it, I started feeling dizzy.

Really dizzy.

(A sign, I now know, of dehydration.)

I began pleading with God: "Please, please, *please*, don't let me faint. I'm so close ..."

After the longest fifteen minutes of my life, I passed the twenty-five-mile marker and realized I could *walk* in and still qualify for Boston. Even so, I didn't relax until I crossed the finish line in 3:22.

An EMT saw me stumbling toward my wife and approached me. "Are you OK? Do you need some help?"

"That's just how he gets," Lisa said, taking my arm. "But he did just qualify for Boston."

"Congratulations!" the guy exclaimed with a big grin.

In spite of my weariness, I managed a smile in return.

Five years. Five marathons. Thousands of miles.

Finally, I had my ticket to Boston.

A Greater Race

"But you, man of God, flee from all this, and *pursue* righteousness, godliness, faith, love, endurance and gentleness."

Perhaps because of my long pursuit of Boston, when I read of Paul's urging Timothy to pursue something, I know what a guy is willing to go through if he wants to pursue something badly enough.

But will I ever pursue righteousness, godliness, faith, love, gentleness, and endurance with the same passion — or more — that I pursued Boston?

Will any of us?

Without becoming critical, think about this honestly: in your own home church, how many Christians fulfill Paul's admonition to truly pursue holiness and Christlikeness?

How many of us who deal with a bad temper ultimately give up and then give in, saying, "That's just the way I am"?

How many have let our bodies decline because we've tried before, maybe on and off for most of our lives, to choose healthier habits, but have concluded that the race can't be won?

How many addicts have made a home in their addiction and are tired of feeling like a failure and unwilling to face another defeat — so they just stop fighting?

There are issues of disobedience in my life that stick to me like superglue. I may have victory over them for months or more, but then the right conditions come back—and *wham!* I think to myself, "Again? Really?"

For instance, there is a certain set of circumstances in my life that, if they happen, I'll usually respond by eating for two days straight, almost without realizing it. The more I eat, the more I *want* to eat. I think I'm opening the barn door just a crack for one tiny indulgence, but it's like throwing wide the gates and getting run over by a herd. Eating *can* make us feel better emotionally, and I've had my share of letting go in that direction.

It would be easy to get discouraged and say, "Real holiness just isn't possible," but Paul speaks to me—and you—when he tells us to pursue holiness. You don't pursue something that isn't elusive. You don't have to! The very notion of pursuit assumes that it takes concerted and repeated effort. Indeed, included in Paul's list is an exaltation of *endurance* itself.

Six hundred years ago, Richard Rolle encouraged believers with words that are as true today as they were then: "Every just man fights immorality and physical desires throughout his life; bad men do not fight at all except against God ... They make a truce with sin."[1]

Our theology—our belief in what is possible—must not be shaped by our *experience* but rather by God's Word. Even if we keep failing in a specific area, Scripture is clear: we need to keep pursuing godliness. For some issues, particularly with eating and exercise, that pursuit may take us eighty years or more. But this doesn't mean we can ever stop running.

Meet My Friend Morty

Because we have positional holiness in the finished work of Jesus Christ, it's tempting to ignore the call to pursue an experiential holiness, which Paul clearly calls us to do in 1 Timothy 6:11.

The fact is, as I've already stated, some sins are extremely difficult to get rid of, and on some level, we will be tempted by certain personally familiar sins until the day we die. We can rise above being enslaved by them, but we may never rise above being enticed by them. We can manage them and gain mastery over them, but we may still be occasionally tripped up by them. How often we are tripped up, however, often depends on our vigilance and effort in fighting back.

Many people give up because they have been lied to. They think they can be cured, rise above the temptation, and never face it (or fall into it) again. Paul wouldn't call us to endurance if God delivered us once and for all whenever we asked him to.

In the face of this imperfect reality, rather than permitting us to just give up, the ancients and Scripture urge Christians to take an active view of pursuing holiness. We can and even *must* cooperate in fighting sin. One of John Baillie's* morning prayers is brilliant: "Let me leave no height of duty behind me unattempted, nor any evil habit unassaulted."[2] Rather than simply wait for sin to attack, Baillie urges us to attack it.

---

* John Baillie (1886–1960) was a Scottish theologian and pastor whose book *A Diary of Private Prayer* is justifiably regarded as a modern devotional classic.

We do this, first, by going on the offensive. Being diligent to go about kingdom business—that's what it means to leave no height of duty unattempted. Second, if we are to leave no evil habit unassaulted, we must fortify ourselves against the allure of sin. The Puritans used the language of mortification—"killing sin"—to express this thought, so let me give a number of contemporary explanations of how modern mortification might take place. If you want a catchy sermon title, you could call this "Making Friends with Morty" (mortification). Notice how each one of these can be helpful tools in fighting what the ancients called "gluttony" and "sloth."

Taste the Bitterness of Your Sin

I love the way John Baillie models how we should address our sin in an evening prayer:

> I remember with bitterness the duties I have shirked:
> I remember with sorrow the hard words I have
>   spoken:
> I remember with shame the unworthy thoughts
>   I have harboured.
> Use these memories, O God, to save me, and then
>   for ever blot them out.[3]

Instead of just dismissing his failings, Baillie wants to first remember them, consider their bitterness, ask God to use the memory of their bitterness to "save" him —i.e., fortify him against such future failings—and then rightly cast himself on God's mercy: "And then for ever blot them out."

Beautiful!

I want to remember how ashamed I was when I finished my *venti* chai before my daughter drank half of her *tall* coffee.

"You're done?" she asked. "Already?"

Next time, Lord, can I at least *taste* it?

I want to remember how awful it felt to drive so impatiently, how ashamed I'd be if someone I knew saw the lack of grace I displayed behind the wheel, and I want to consider what it did to my blood pressure and how it made me forget all about God and how that's not the kind of person I want to be, even though I am that person more often than I'd like to admit.

"Use these memories, O God, to save me, and then for ever blot them out."

Examine the Deceit behind the Sin

Sin, in its stark-naked reality, essentially calls God a liar: "Your way isn't the best way. You want to deny me something that is good. You're misleading me as to how I should live." The reason we need to look at our rebellion in all its ugliness is so that our thinking can be changed. Paul says we are transformed by the renewing of our minds (Romans 12:2).

What this means is that every point of sin is a point of disagreement with God. And when we disagree with God, guess who is in the wrong? When we sin, we're telling God, explicitly or implicitly, "You say to live this way, but I think it's better to live that way."

Go back to that moment of temptation and ask

yourself, *When, exactly, did I begin to call God a liar?* Do you see how you were deceived?

Did opening the bag of chips, even though your conscience was telling you not to, really help you feel better thirty minutes later, or did you feel worse? Did blowing off the exercise session — even though, many times before, exercising when you didn't feel like it made you feel renewed and invigorated — serve your long-term goal of better health? Or was it simply a matter of coddling a soft spirit? There are times when it's wise and even necessary to skip working out, but was this one of them?

By thinking this through carefully, you are renewing your mind and preparing yourself for the next assault. Don't just accept the deceit. In the calm of grace and forgiveness, with God as your loving physician and teacher, reexamine the deceit so you begin to understand where and how you were deceived, and then fortify yourself with God's truth so that you won't be fooled by the same deceit the next time. At least make Satan come up with a new lie! Thinking through your failings will remind you just how much of a liar Satan and our own desires can be.

Consider the Circumstances of Your Sin

Third, we need to consider the circumstances of our sin. Spend some time asking yourself why you were so vulnerable. Does this sin assault you when you feel tired, ashamed, lonely, afraid, frustrated? Can you discern any common circumstances that set you up for such a fall?

If so, you can anticipate those circumstances and seek to prepare for them ahead of time. If you always overeat in the afternoon, consider scheduling walks with a friend. If you consistently lose your temper at a certain point in the week, talk with your spouse about trying to find a way to ease the pressure before you get to that point. There was a time in my life when I routinely overate by snacking after dinner. I looked at the circumstances, the common patterns, and changed them by adjusting my schedule and adopting spot fasting.

In other words, after we've sinned, let's remember that there is work to be done, not to earn forgiveness and merit God's renewed favor and acceptance, but to fortify our souls against future falls of the same kind.

Use the Exposure That Sin Provides to Gain a More Accurate View of the Condition of Your Soul

One "blessing" of sin (if we can ever call it that) is that it can usher us into a new honesty. Our frailty is exposed, and we have the opportunity to say, "I think I'm afraid about ... [or ashamed or more tired than I realized or frustrated, and so forth]." If we rush right to forgiveness, we will miss the value of "living in the light"—i.e., being completely honest with ourselves.

When Charlie Weiss took over as head coach of the

Notre Dame football team, he told his players (referring to their previous season), "Here's the reality: you're a 6 and 5 football team. That's not good enough for you, and it's not good enough for me."

The fact that they wore the colors of Notre Dame didn't change the fact that their actions on the field made them an average 6 and 5 team. (Which is why when Weiss's team went 6 and 6, he was fired!)

I may call myself a Christian, and I may wear my faith on my sleeve, but if I talk about others behind their back, I'm a gossip. If I treat my wife harshly, I'm mean. If I fail to train my kids, I'm lazy. That's what I am.

Let your sin tell you what you are so that you can reclaim what God has made you to be — a pursuer of righteousness, godliness, faith, love, endurance, and gentleness.

Consider the Strength of Your Sin

How strong is this sin that seeks to take you down? Have you been gaining victory over it, or has the sin been gaining victory over you? Is it becoming more or less common? If its power is growing, you need to be appropriately concerned and seek out help. Don't let a particular sin gain mastery over you. Be honest and vigilant here. Is this a somewhat unusual "sin of passion," responding to the moment, or is it a growing habit? If a sin is consistently getting the best of you, it's time to seek help. Bringing it into the light through confession and accountability can kill it before it kills you.

Find a Holy Substitute

Next, consider a pure alternative to this sin. One of my main goals in my previous book, *Pure Pleasure*, is to help us see how God can use appropriate pleasure to fortify our souls.[4] If you find yourself giving in to negative gossip, can you build some friendships in which conversation is enriching and gossip isn't tolerated? If you consistently sin while you're traveling, is there a good activity on the road that can replace this sin?

I know of a famous baseball player who was a Christian when called up to the big leagues. He was a married man who was well aware of the potential for sin both inside and outside Major League Baseball locker rooms. It wasn't the lifestyle he wanted to lead, so he began playing video games in his hotel room. He knew he was going to be gone from home for more than a hundred nights a year. Simply gritting his teeth and trying to repress temptation night after night wouldn't work. He needed to find an acceptable alternative, something he could look forward to when his teammates went out drinking, clubbing, and worse. For him, it was video games.

I had always thought of video games as somewhat wasteful entertainment at best—until I heard this story. God bless him for earnestly desiring to stay true to his faith and his marriage in a world of temptation.

If eating is your issue, many therapists wisely recommend taking spontaneity out of the equation. A lot of overeating happens on the spur of the moment. To counteract this, write out what you're going to eat and stick to your schedule. On Monday, you have oatmeal and toast for breakfast, a turkey sandwich on pita bread for lunch, an afternoon snack of yogurt and almonds, and a chicken salad for dinner. On Tuesday, something else — and so on. Let the food schedule be your protector. Let it end all argument ("No, that's not what I'm eating — I'm eating *this*").

Instead of giving in and eating half a cheesecake, find some dark chocolate you really enjoy and take your time to cherish each bite. See how long you can make the sensible-sized piece last. If you know you're going to eat *something* for dessert, decide in advance on a reasonable portion. Prepare for the onslaught with an acceptable substitute.

Fortify Your Soul

Finally, consider how you can fortify your soul with spiritual enrichment. There are sermons and books on virtually every issue a Christian might face. Meditating on Scripture is powerfully effective. The spiritual disciplines, such as fasting, solitude, meditation, and the like, can be very helpful. The Puritans called the Sabbath the "market day of the soul." It's a day we work on our holiness — but don't restrict this exercise to one day. Why not listen to several sermons a week? Why not read from the Scriptures and the classics on a daily basis?

Olympic athletes have daily workouts; what's your

daily *spiritual* workout? What are you doing to become stronger, wiser, more mature?

The point of "making friends with Morty" is to avoid falling into the trap of thinking that saying, "I'm sorry, God" marks the end of our role in pursuing holiness. This is lazy spirituality. It's not walking in grace—it's walking in laziness. You know this is true. Be honest. Has this approach ever even lessened the occurrence of sin in your life? Take the time and make the effort to fight sin with the tools God provides.

Physical Acts, Spiritual Consequences

Let me connect some of my earlier reflections about physical fitness to this battle against spiritual laziness. We grow into holiness like we grow into fitness. As a believer, Jim Ryun applied the physical lessons about training for the mile to his spiritual life:

> I didn't just roll out of bed one morning and say, "I'm lacing up my shoes, stepping out the door and running a sub-four-minute mile." My rise began first with a goal. Then came a plan, step by step how I was going to achieve my goal. It took a focus previously unknown to me. But the road to success was not without bumps. There were injuries, delays and incredible physical and mental exhaustion.[5]

Laziness would have killed this goal, just like it kills so many New Year's resolutions. But Ryun persevered.

> We all yearn for spiritual growth, but we want the quick fix; we want it all now. But just as I had to keep training as a young runner, putting one foot in front of the other in that icy weather, we have to discipline ourselves spiritually, putting one foot in front of the other to move toward the upward calling of Christ Jesus. It takes discipline, and it takes time. But it also takes ownership.[6]

When addressing eating and exercise, the same principles apply. There may not be a quick fix. You'll have to set goals, gradually build up your spirit, and persevere. The ungodly fail once and often give up trying, but living with God's grace gives us the strength to persevere in the face of repeated failure.

The payoff goes far beyond "not doing something." Holiness, a life and character of love, and a godly demeanor have a big reward—just as physical training can.

April 2009

It felt like a dream.

The Porta-Potty lines were long, but the crowd was jovial, energized, electric. Everyone here was used to this. Everyone here, in one sense, wouldn't have it any other way, as most of us tended toward the obsessive-compulsive personality trait.

"Is this your first one?" the sixty-year-old man asked me.

"Yes."

He and his buddy, the same age, slapped each other's shoulders and smiled knowingly.

"Are you going to cry?" he asked me.

"I really don't know."

"Well, don't be embarrassed if you do. I've done six of these, and I've cried every time."

Forty-five minutes later, I found out why.

Leaving the athletes' village, tens of thousands of runners walked three-quarters of a mile to one of the most hallowed places of ground among runners: the start of the Boston marathon.

The first brush with emotion occurred when the official let me into my carrel, reserved for those with numbers 9000 to 9999 on their chest.

He let me in, I thought. *He let me in*.

The second occurred when the fighter jets flew overhead, and people started murmuring.

The third happened when the gun went off, and over 8,000 runners preceded me for the start of the marathon, with another 16,000 runners behind me.

The fourth happened when my feet crossed the official starting line, more than seven minutes later. Families were yelling, shaking noisemakers, holding up signs, clapping their hands.

I got to see all the landmarks (and a surprising number of Dunkin' Donuts franchises)—including the "screaming tunnel" around Wellesley College, Heart-break Hill, and the famous Citgo sign along Common-wealth Avenue, which marks one mile to go.

I'll never forget finally turning left on Boylston Street, thousands of people *still* screaming as we made our way toward the finish line and the last two hundred meters of the race. Up to that point, I hadn't shed a single tear, but I could imagine how anyone else might, including two sixty-year-old buddies running together.

I thought of the effort required in taking a forty-something body—made soft by life, by a desk job, by raising young children—and getting it to travel 26.2 miles in time to qualify for Boston; the five all-out attempts, months of miles, years of black toenails, body parts bleeding that you wouldn't normally think of as capable of bleeding, running on the road in strange places and sometimes horrendous weather, bottles of ibuprofen and gallons of ice, desperately searching for out-of-the-way Porta-Potties during the middle of long runs, being in an unfamiliar town and just as desper-ately looking for a water fountain or convenience store on a sweltering day.

But it was the difficulty, the pain, the frequent failure, that made the two-hundred-meter jaunt down Boylston Street all the more meaningful and cherished. If the pursuit had been easy, there wouldn't have been half the joy in finishing the race.

I looked up, the blue and yellow Boston finish ban-ner growing closer by the step, and lifted my head and pointed at the sky, acknowledging the Creator who made this possible.

That's when I started to cry.

The day will come when you and I will see a very different "finish line." My father-in-law saw that line just months ago, when he was only hours away from leaving this world. He could see his deceased father, and he saw the Lord's hands: "His hands, his hands," he said. "Help me slide into his hands."

Such a day will come for each one of us—we will be but minutes away from entering eternity. On that day, our frequent defeats, our never-ending struggles, all our efforts, will only make the fact that we can slide into those marked hands all the sweeter. We can't earn our way there; we'll enter by the marks on *his* hands, not ours. But we'll be glad we persevered. We'll be glad we can say with Paul, "I have fought the good fight, I have finished the race, I have kept the faith. Now there is in store for me the crown of righteousness, which the Lord, the righteous Judge, will award to me on that day —and not only to me, but also to all who have longed for his appearing" (2 Timothy 4:7–8).

15

THE LAST CHRISTIAN

The T-ball player connected with the baseball, launching a white missile that stopped only when it hit my six-year-old son's forehead.

Graham dropped like he had been hit by a sledgehammer. I ran out to the infield, next to the coach. "Are you all right, bud?" I asked.

Graham nodded his head. "I think so."

I could already see the knot forming just above his left eye. Graham started to get up, and the coach said, "Here, we'll help you off the field and put Tyler in."

"No," Graham protested. "Tyler lets the balls go by. We can still win this game. I can play."

"Are you sure?" I asked.

"Yeah."

I looked at the coach, who shrugged his shoulders

and said, "Graham's better groggy than Tyler is clear-headed, so if it's OK with you ..."

The coach and I patted Graham on the back, and I returned to the bench, feeling very proud thoughts, saying to myself, "This is so cool; I've got a really *tough* son! Who knew?"

When a kid is just five or six years old, untested, you really don't know, and I couldn't have been happier with life in general until, on my way back to the bench, I caught my wife's gaze.

Visual daggers flew out of her eyes with the force of a hurricane. We had been married long enough for her to know how to yell at me while being totally silent, and she was screaming.

My six-year-old son just got hit in the head with a hard baseball, and you're leaving him out there? Have you lost your mind? What if he has a concussion? What if, now that he's groggy, he gets hit by another ball? Do you realize how despicable you are?

I made the gutless decision to remain on the bench with the coach instead of returning to the bleachers, as I could only imagine the conversation my wife was having with her friends — something along the lines of, "There are three despicable men in the history of the universe: Adolf Hitler, Judas Iscariot, and my husband."

After the game, we had a "discussion," in which we sort of had to agree to disagree. I finally told my wife, "This is not a world in which weak men do well."

"He's a *boy*, Gary," Lisa countered.

"That's right, honey," I said. "He's a *boy*. And I've got to raise him to act like one."

Now that I've undoubtedly angered a number of readers with what might, out of context, sound like a sexist statement, allow me to broaden it across genders: This is not a generation in which weak Christians will do well. With all the challenges facing the contemporary church, we need, as much as anything, to raise tough believers.

All this talk about fitness, facing the pain of getting in shape, actively combating indulgence and laziness, is in many ways an appeal for the church to get tougher. We are soft. We often cave in at the slightest challenge. Men are lost to superficial sins; women are lost to superficial cares, and the work of the kingdom is neglected. If we don't get tougher, the work will never get done.

What if, as he has throughout history, God allows the faithful to be universally persecuted to the point of our becoming isolated, hunted, and scattered? What if, as already is true in many countries, a person had to choose between remaining true to God and being gainfully employed, or even married? Would we still be standing, would we still sign up, if we thought we were the last Christian?

That's an image I want to leave in your mind as we near the end of this book. If you didn't know anyone else who shared your faith; if you were assaulted psychologically, relationally, vocationally, financially, and even physically, would you still make a stand for Jesus?

Until that moment comes, none of us really know

EVERY BODY MATTERS

for sure. But this notion of being "the last Christian" is an image that has borne considerable fruit in my own life as I seek to become the Christian that God wants me to be and the Christian that the church needs each of us to be.

There's a dangerous, elitist element in this question about taking a stand as the last Christian that could lead some to strike out against the church, and that's certainly not my intention. But perhaps if we placed it in the context of Paul's words in 2 Timothy, it becomes helpful. Paul informs his young disciple, "You know that everyone in the province of Asia has deserted me, including Phygelus and Hermogenes"—but then remembers a past saint: "May the Lord show mercy to the household of Onesiphorus, because he often refreshed me and was not ashamed of my chains. On the contrary, when he was in Rome, he searched hard for me until he found me" (1:15–17).

The most natural reading of this passage is that Onesiphorus has died* and Paul feels abandoned and somewhat alone, cherishing memories of a faithful friend who has graduated to glory.

---

* Commentators debate this, in part because of the historical controversy in which some Roman Catholic commentators argued for Onesiphoros's death in order to support offering prayers for the dead, which led many Protestants to argue against it so as to refute such a practice. The most natural reading seems to be that Paul is thinking back on a faithful friend who has left this world. New Testament scholar Dr. Gordon Fee takes this position in his commentary on 1 and 2 Timothy and Titus in the New International Biblical Commentary series.

In this context, we can ask ourselves, if an entire area were to slowly abandon the faith, would we be a Hermogenes or an Onesiphoros? Would we not only refuse to abandon God's servants who speak the truth, but would we actively seek them out to provide encouragement and support in Jesus' name?

Such a commitment will require radical spiritual strength, and I believe that addressing the physical issues of laziness and overeating can have a significant impact on the church's readiness. I don't believe that riding a bike for a hundred miles, swimming across a lake, or running a marathon counts as "carrying our cross," but getting in shape can help us build souls *willing* to carry a cross.

Listen to the wise words of Lorenzo Scupoli:

> If any employment is irksome to you, either on its own account, or because of the person who laid it on you; or, if you dislike it because it hinders you from doing what you like better, still undertake it and complete it, whatever trouble it may be to you, and though you might find comfort by not doing it. If you leave it, you will never learn to suffer, and true peace will never be your portion, because it does not spring except from a soul purified from passion and adorned with holiness.[1]

Scupoli wisely urges us to use discomfort to train our souls, suggesting (correctly) that a spirit of surrender and sacrifice isn't accidental or passively cultivated, but rather springs from an intentional life of devotion and pursuit. Doesn't this put our daily battles of physical fitness in an entirely new light? How many times have we stood on the precipice of choosing between exercising or eating a plate of nachos? Maybe it's raining outside, and we don't like the thought of getting wet. Perhaps we just "feel" like lying down and watching television instead of getting on the StairMaster while we watch. We can skip the exercise and indulge our stomachs, or we can grow in grace, strength, and spiritual vitality. Such common, seemingly trivial physical tests have huge spiritual implications.

"Pain Unending ... Grievous and Incurable"

When the church looks for examples of extreme toughness, it should consider the life of the Old Testament prophet Jeremiah. All that Jeremiah had to endure during a public ministry that lasted for about forty years is enough to frighten the bravest saint.

Early in his life, the call to become a prophet looked like a relatively convenient one: Jeremiah began his prophetic work under the reign of Josiah, a God-fearing leader who initiated radical reforms and turned an entire nation back to God. Twelve years later, however, Josiah died, and the bottom fell out for Jeremiah. King Jehoiakim cowered under Babylon's gluttonous consumption of the Middle East, and in his fear he turned to idols. Jeremiah soon found himself at odds with the entire leadership of Israel—religious *and* political

—and even his own family betrayed him (12:6). By standing up for God and against idolatry, he was called a traitor. The persecution was so intense and painful that Jeremiah described it as "my pain unending . . . my wound grievous and incurable" (15:18).

When Jeremiah nevertheless continued to faithfully proclaim God's words, even to an increasingly hostile audience, the chief priest of God's temple had him beaten and put in stocks (20:1–2). When Jeremiah *still* chose obedience to God over people pleasing, all the religious leaders gathered and told the political leaders and citizens of Israel, "This man should be sentenced to death" (26:11).

By God's providence, Jeremiah lived to see another day, but he certainly never became a bestselling author or a popular speaker on the religious circuit. In fact, on one occasion, as Jeremiah wrote down prophetic words from God and had them delivered to the king, Jehoiakim simply burned the words of the scroll as they were read (Jeremiah 36). Jeremiah's masterpiece didn't even make it into a second printing!

Jehoiakim died, as did his son after a very short reign, and then Jeremiah had to prophesy under one of the most pathetic, weak-willed, mealy mouthed leaders you could ever imagine—King Zedekiah. Imagine every United States president's worst weakness, without any president's primary strengths, put them in one person, and you'd have Zedekiah.

Zedekiah asks Jeremiah to pray for him and the nation, but after Jeremiah prophesies, Zedekiah has

him arrested on his way home on a trumped-up political charge. Jeremiah's prison is disgustingly brutal, a
dungeon, and Jeremiah is kept there, in the words of
Scripture, "a long time" (37:16). When Zedekiah finally
brings Jeremiah back out, we get a sense of just how
awful the prison must have been, as Jeremiah makes
a special plea: "Do not send me back ... or I will die
there" (37:20). Zedekiah relents, allows Jeremiah to be
held in a prison courtyard, and orders that he be given
a loaf of bread each day (who knows what he was eating before ...).

Think about it: called to a public ministry, betrayed
by your own family and the religious rulers, considered
a traitor by your government, truly standing alone, persecuted for your faithfulness. Who among us wouldn't
grow bitter at such treatment? Who among us, indeed,
would ever think of developing a prosperity gospel out
of such a life?

Yet Jeremiah's struggles had just begun.

Some local officials pleaded with Zedekiah to put
Jeremiah to death. The weak-willed king couldn't say
no to anyone: "He is in your hands ... The king can
do nothing to oppose you" (38:5). The officials then
lowered Jeremiah into a cistern—a covered recepta-
cle used to store water. Imagine being lowered into a
narrow well that is dark at the bottom, with no fresh
air. This particular cistern had no water in it, but the
bottom was likely covered in mud or muck. Jeremiah
could have been standing waist-deep in a stinking bog,

surrounded by darkness and who knows what kind of insects, filth, and stench.

Another official eventually takes pity on Jeremiah and pleads with Zedekiah to release him. The king, quite predictably, goes along (he can't say no to anyone), and it takes thirty men to tug Jeremiah off the muddy floor and raise him back onto dry ground, but Jeremiah is still held in captivity.

Zedekiah visits him in secret, makes Jeremiah promise to lie about why the king was visiting him, and yet still fails to take Jeremiah's counsel. As much as we like to complain about our leaders today, we haven't yet had to endure a Zedekiah, whose actions and inactions ultimately led to the destruction of Jerusalem and the captivity of its inhabitants.

In the end, Jeremiah's warnings failed. He and his fellow Israelites were carted off into exile. If you measured Jeremiah's anointing and stature by any standard used for Christian celebrities today, he would be considered an absolute, total failure.

How discouraging all of this must have been to a prophet who remained faithful in spite of some of the worst abuse ever endured by one of God's servants.

The Last One

Here is my point in recounting Jeremiah's story in the context of talking about "the last Christian": Who among us today would have the strength, the perseverance, the courage, to live such a life and endure such a ministry? A weak man or woman, expecting nothing but prosperity, comfort, and health, would wilt within two weeks. Isn't it likely that a prophet who is prone to overeating would cave in the face of such utter deprivation? A soft body cannot carry a hard message; a fragile personality cannot endure a harsh response.

Consider also the case of the apostle Paul. He could not have been a weak man. We're told in Acts 14 that while in Lystra, Paul was pelted with stones, dragged outside the city, and left for dead. If *his persecutors* thought he was dead, Paul must have been pretty beat-up. Yet we're also told that after they left him, Paul got up and went back into the city, and "the next day he and Barnabas left for Derbe" (verse 20). The next day! For the record, Derbe was over *sixty miles* from Lystra. A physically weak man could never have recovered like that.

To the Corinthians, Paul wrote of a ministry that is astonishingly difficult: "As servants of God we commend ourselves in every way: in great endurance; in troubles, hardships and distresses; in beatings, imprisonments and riots; in hard work, sleepless nights and hunger ..." (2 Corinthians 6:4–5). How could a lazy glutton ever live up to a life like this? Paul endured hunger, long hours, and physical pain, heaped on each other like the layers of lasagna that show up at every church potluck. Let's think about that the next time we wonder why the church has gone so soft.

It is the church's duty and calling to raise men and women with the strength of Jeremiah and Paul who will not wilt in the face of the fiercest persecution imaginable. In the annals of Christian history, I think of the condescension and ever-present threat of excommunication and even death under which the spiritual stalwart Teresa of Avila carried out her mission, or the devastating disfigurement and social ostracism endured by Jeanne Guyon.

I can barely describe some of the horrendous, personally hurtful e-mails that contemporary leaders such as Rick and Kay Warren, Beth Moore, Ed Young, and others endure on almost a daily basis. Even J. I. Packer has been threatened by his denomination with ecclesiastical censure for courageously maintaining a biblical stand that is in line with Scripture's clear teaching and with what the church has accepted for thousands of years.

Friends, if they're coming for J. I. Packer, eventually they're coming for us!

We know we have grown soft. Many if not most of us, simply could not last in the face of such social or physical challenges. Becoming spiritually and physically fit are two ways that we can grow in our inner and outer strength, as well as in our ability and willingness to endure hardship. The end result is that we, like Jeremiah and Paul, may become truly useful to the Master and prepared to do any good work.

In the inspiring words of Johannes Tauler:

Whenever one finds such men or women, one finds nothing but divine life. Their conduct, their actions, their whole manner of life is divinized. They are noble souls, and the whole of Christendom draws profit from them. To all they give sustenance, to God glory, and to humankind consolation. They dwell in God, and God in them. Wherever they are they should be praised. May God grant that we, too, may have a share in this.[2]

EPILOGUE

> In a large house there are articles not only of gold and silver, but also of wood and clay; some are for special purposes and some for common use. Those who cleanse themselves from the latter will be instruments for special purposes, made holy, useful to the Master and prepared to do any good work.
>
> 2 Timothy 2:20–21

Before I had even met him and benefited from having him as my adviser, Dr. J. I. Packer challenged me as a college student when he wrote that people who love God attempt great things for him. The famous evangelist Dwight Moody had a similar mind-set on his deathbed when he told his sons, "If God be your partner, let your plans be large."

How can we embrace godly ambition as well as the

universal call to a humble spirit proclaimed by Scripture and virtually every worthy Christian classic? In humility, we recognize we can do nothing on our own; and Christ's love compels us to reach out beyond what is possible in our own strength. This is a cooperative work. Humility is the friend of spiritual ambition, not its foe. Lazy passivity isn't humility; it is laziness masquerading as a spiritual virtue.

Read through the Gospels with fresh eyes, and you may be amazed at how much Jesus could pack into a *single* day.

Pick up a copy of John Wesley's journal. You'll read the account of a man who preached several times a day, wrote something for the printer at least once every week, and who traveled by horseback from town to town, many times in the rain and always on the back roads, through bogs, wilderness, and difficult country, to proclaim the gospel. His was a tireless life of service. I defy you not to become exhausted merely *reading* about his exploits.

Take up a biography of Teresa of Avila, whose passion to reform lapsed convents and monasteries led her to work and travel tirelessly in the face of much opposition and even persecution, despite her own ill health and physical infirmities.

Then pick up a biography of Henry Drummond, a Scottish leader in the early YMCA movement and a close associate of Dwight Moody. He organized and held three group meetings *a day*, each of which was followed by earnest one-on-one encounters with seekers and new converts. Drummond wisely taught, "Each life should be a mission."[1]

Yes, of course there is a place for rest, Sabbath, and vacation—encased within a life of diligent work. In the midst of that, let us exalt the life championed by Theodore Roosevelt:

> The credit belongs to the man who is actually in the arena, whose face is marred by dust and sweat and blood; who strives valiantly; who errs, who comes short again and again, because there is no effort without error and shortcoming; but who does actually strive to do the deeds; who knows the great enthusiasms, the great devotions; who spends himself in a worthy cause; who at the best knows in the end the triumph of high achievement, and who at the worst, if he fails, at least fails while daring greatly, so that his place shall never be with those cold and timid souls who know neither victory nor defeat.[2]

Isn't this the kind of life we should all aspire to live, as God provides the ability and strength to do so? Let's seek to embrace, within a Christian context, the life experience described by a friend of ultramarathoner Dean Karnazes: "Life is not a journey to the grave with the intention of arriving safely in a pretty and well-preserved body, but rather to skid in broadside, thoroughly used up, totally worn out, and loudly proclaiming: 'WOW!! What a ride!'"[3]

A Final Vision

I am not, by nature, a particularly mystical sort of person. I'm far more studious and cognitive. But there was one prayer time that, in spite of my hesitancy, provided a vision for my future that I believe sets up the perfect ending for this study.

I had just completed a somewhat exhausting weekend doing a seminar and then giving the Sunday sermons at a church. All this came at the end of what had already been a long week, with much work ahead in the coming week, and I was very tired. I also felt a bit discouraged, wondering if all this effort was producing any fruit. My books were hanging in there, but they weren't breaking out and becoming conversation starters, as the publisher had hoped.

The vision had me running along a mountainous pass. It was rainy and windy, and the sky was dark — and getting darker. I came across a mountain cabin of some sort and was welcomed in by Jesus himself. It's somewhat startling that I wasn't surprised to "see" Jesus, but I guess that's the way these things go.

I was muddy, soaked, bloody, sore, and tired — obviously from being on a very long run. Jesus welcomed me in and beckoned me to sit in a chair. I was given a warm drink and something to eat. The energy boost was immediate — astonishingly so. Jesus removed my wet shoes and socks and replaced them with dry ones — what a luxury to wear dry socks and shoes! He then removed my shirt and gave me a dry one — it felt like heaven itself to take off a damp, sweaty, rain-soaked shirt and wear something soft and dry.

As I finished the drink and the bread, Jesus bandaged up some bleeding cuts and scrapes on my legs. I felt like a new man. Jesus then looked in my eyes, stood up, and said some wonderful things I will not share.

I was feeling so affirmed, warm, and cozy, when Jesus hugged me and pointed toward the door, now suddenly open. I could see that it was still raining, and the wind was still howling. It was getting even darker. Jesus gently placed his hand on my back and said, "Now, Gary, *keep running.*"

I went back out into the rain, a new man with a new desire and renewed strength.

As I write this, my race isn't over. I don't know how long it will last. Maybe it'll be finished tomorrow. Maybe next year, or several decades hence. God alone knows. But this much I do know: If you're reading this, your race isn't over either. God will restore us and refresh us along the way. He will provide moments of nourishment and rest, but he wants me, he wants you, to continue to run, to be available to do any good work. We need to keep going—even in the rain, no matter how dark it gets—and finish this race.

Christian, *keep running.*

ACKNOWLEDGMENTS

I'm thankful to John Sloan and Dirk Buursma for their typical editing prowess; Mike Salisbury and Tom Dean for getting excited about a book that others raised their eyebrows at; my agent, Curtis Yates, whom I grow to be more thankful for every day; and the entire team at Zondervan for a ten-year partnership in the gospel.

In addition to my gratitude to those who allowed themselves to be interviewed and quoted in this book, I express thanks to those who read and provided comments on early drafts, including: Mary Kay Smith, Steve and Candice Watters, Deb Steinkamp, Laurie Prall, Virginia Knowles, Erik Johnson, Jim Schmotzer, Paul Petersen, Mark Warren, Bruce Becker, Randy Pries, Bill Palmer, Tom Beaumont, and Dr. Nick Yphantides. No single reader agreed with every comment contained in this book, but the interplay that resulted from wrestling through these issues proved immensely fruitful for me and, I hope, will be equally fruitful for future readers.

NOTES

CHAPTER 1: Souls of Silver

1. Ed Young, Jo Beth Young, Michael Duncan, Richard Leachman, *Total Heart Health for Men: A Life-Enriching Plan for Physical and Spiritual Well-Being* (Nashville: Nelson, 2007), 166.

CHAPTER 2: Heads without Bodies

1. Elton Trueblood, *The Common Ventures of Life* (New York: Harper, 1949), 16.

2. Carolyn Arends, "Matter Matters," *Christianity Today* 53 (August 2009): 52, www.christianitytoday.com/ct/2009/august/13.52.html?start=1 (January 6, 2011).

3. Quoted in Kenneth Cooper, *Faith-Based Fitness* (Nashville: Nelson, 1995), 25.

4. Ibid., 63.

5. William Law, *A Serious Call to a Devout and Holy Life* (1729; repr., New York: Paulist, 1978), 216–17.

6. Ed Young, Jo Beth Young, Michael Duncan, Richard Leachman, 365 *Days of Total Heart Health: Transform Your Physical and Spiritual Life* (Nashville: Nelson, 2005), 14.

CHAPTER 3: "Your Strength Will Equal Your Days"

1. David A. Kessler, *The End of Overeating: Taking Control of the Insatiable American Appetite* (New York: Rodale, 2009), 7.

2. Ed Young, Jo Beth Young, Michael Duncan, Richard Leachman, *Total Heart Health for Men: A Life-Enriching Plan for Physical and Spiritual Well-Being* (Nashville: Nelson, 2007), 41.

3. Ibid.

4. Dr. Kenneth H. Cooper, *Faith-Based Fitness* (Nashville: Nelson, 1995), 7.

5. Ibid.

6. John Calvin, *Institutes of the Christian Religion*, ed. John T. McNeill (1559; repr., Philadelphia: Westminster, 1960), 1.705 – 6.

7. Young, Young, Duncan, and Leachman, *Total Heart Health for Men*, 41.

CHAPTER 4: Healthy Humiliation

1. Dr. Kenneth H. Cooper, *Faith-Based Fitness* (Nashville: Nelson, 1995), 12.

2. Ibid., 219.

3. Ibid., 222.

4. Haruki Murakami, *What I Talk About When I Talk About Running* (New York: Knopf, 2008), 42.

5. Dietrich Bonhoeffer, *The Cost of Discipleship*, trans. R. H. Fuller (New York: Macmillan, 1963), 189.

6. Kristin Armstrong, foreword to *Running—The Sacred Art: Preparing to Practice*, by Warren A. Kay (Woodstock, Vt.: SkyLight Paths, 2007), xi.

CHAPTER 5: **It's Not a Fair Fight**

1. The 1997 National Health Interview Survey, cited in R. Marie Griffith, *Born Again Bodies: Flesh and Spirit in American Christianity* (Los Angeles: University of California Press, 2004), 230.

2. An insightful paper by John DelHousaye, "Would Jesus Eat a Whopper (with Cheese)?" (presented at the sixtieth annual meeting of the Evangelical Theological Society on November 20, 2008), inspired some of the thoughts and provided the background for these points, which I've restated in this section.

3. David A. Kessler, *The End of Overeating* (New York: Rodale, 2009), 69.

4. Quoted in ibid., 125.

5. Ibid., 139.

6. Ibid., 140.

7. Nanci Hellmich, "Portion Sizes Increase in 'Last Supper' Paintings," *USA Today*, March 23, 2010, 11B, www.usatoday.com/news/health/weightloss/2010-03-23-last supper23_ST_N.htm (January 5, 2011).

CHAPTER 6: **Is Being Overweight a Sin?**

1. John Chrysostom, "Homily on Philippians 14.3.18–21," cited in *Ancient Christian Commentary on Scripture, New Testament: Galatians, Ephesians, Philippians*, ed. Mark Edwards (Downers Grove, Ill.: InterVarsity, 1999), 8:263.

2. John Chrysostom, "Homilies on the Epistles of Paul to the Corinthians 17.1," cited in *Ancient Christian Commentary on Scripture, New Testament: 1, 2 Corinthians*, ed. Gerald Bray (Downers Grove, Ill.: InterVarsity, 1999), 7:55.

3. Jerome, "Against Jovinian 2:7," cited in *The Great Sayings of Jesus: Proverbs, Parables and Prayers*, ed. John Drane (New York: St. Martin's, 1999), 53.

4. John Climacus, *The Ladder of Divine Ascent*, trans. Colm Luibheid and Norman Russell (New York: Paulist, 1982), 168–69.

5. Ibid., 106.

6. Ibid., 159.

7. Ibid., 168.

8. François Fénelon, *Christian Perfection*, trans. Mildred Whitney Stillman (Minneapolis: Bethany House, 1975), 35.

9. Dietrich Bonhoeffer, *The Cost of Discipleship*, trans. R. H. Fuller (New York: Macmillan, 1963), 188.

10. William Law, *A Serious Call to a Devout and Holy Life* (New York: Paulist, 1978), 191–92.

11. Climacus, *Ladder of Divine Ascent*, 133.

12. See R. Marie Griffith, *Born Again Bodies* (Los Angeles: University of California Press, 2004), 42.

13. John Wesley, *Sermons on Several Occasions* (Leeds: Edward Baines, 1799), 363.

14. Henry Drummond, *The Ideal Life and Other Unpublished Addresses* (1899; repr., New York: Kessinger, 2003), 264.

15. Ibid., 264–65.

CHAPTER 7: Socially Contagious

1. Nicholas Christakis [professor of medical sociology at Harvard Medical School] and James Fowler [professor of political science at University of California, San Diego], "The Spread of Obesity in a Large Social Network over 32 Years," *New England Journal of Medicine* 357 (July 26, 2007): 370–79.

2. Scott VanLue, with Tom Gill, *Does Health Care, Do You Care?* (Columbus, Ga.: TEC Publications, 2005), 7.

3. Cited in R. Marie Griffith, *Born Again Bodies* (Los Angeles: University of California Press, 2004), 2–3.

CHAPTER 8: The Silent Murderer

1. Julian of Norwich, *Revelations of Divine Love*, trans. Elizabeth Spearing (New York: Penguin, 1998), 107.

2. Quoted in Ugolino di Monte Santa Maria, *The Little Flowers of Saint Francis*, trans. Raphael Brown (New York: Image, 1958), 270.

3. Richard Rolle, *The English Writings*, trans. Rosamund Allen (New York: Paulist, 1988), 70.

4. Johannes Tauler, *Sermons*, trans. Maria Shrady (New York: Paulist, 1985), 138.

5. Lorenzo Scupoli, *The Spiritual Combat* (1589; repr., Manchester, N.H.: Sophia Institute, 2002), 60.

6. Jac. Müller, *The Epistles of Paul to the Philippians and to Philemon* (1955; repr., Grand Rapids: Eerdmans, 1980), 124.

7. Jonathan Edwards, *Religious Affections*, ed. James Houston (1746; repr., Minneapolis: Bethany House, 1984), 8.

8. Ibid., 168.

9. John Stott, *Guard the Gospel: The Message of 2 Timothy* (Downers Grove, Ill.: InterVarsity, 1973), 57.

10. Scupoli, *Spiritual Combat*, 61.

11. Ibid., 63.

12. Henry Drummond, *The Greatest Thing in the World*, ed. Harold J. Chadwick (1880; repr., Gainesville, Fla.: Bridge-Logos, 2005), 26.

13. Ibid., 26–27.

14. Ibid., 37.

CHAPTER 9: **Let's Get Physical**

1. Dr. Mehmet Oz and Dr. Michael Roizen, "Better Man 2008: Retool, Reboot, Rebuild," *Esquire*, May 2008, 122.

2. Quoted in Dimity McDowell, "Running through the Ages," *Runner's World*, March 2008, 62.

3. Oz and Roizen, "Better Man 2008: Retool, Reboot, Rebuild," 122.

4. Quoted in Nanci Hellmich, "Quality of Life Improves with Exercise," *USA Today*, February 10, 2009, 5D,

www.usatoday.com/news/health/weightloss/2009-02
-09-quality-life-exercise_N.htm (January 6, 2011).

5. See Kathleen Fackelmann, "Author: Regular Workouts 'Spark' Brain," *USA Today*, February 19, 2008, 12D, www.usatoday.com/news/health/2008-02-18-brain -spark_N.htm (January 7, 2011).

6. David A. Kessler, *The End of Overeating* (New York: Rodale, 2009), 224.

7. Quoted in Fackelmann, "Regular Workouts 'Spark' Brain," 12D.

8. Cited in Nanci Hellmich, "Obesity Takes a Health— and Financial—Toll," *USA Today*, December 28, 2009, 4D.

9. David Zinczenko, "Feeding the Obesity Epidemic," *USA Today*, March 25, 2008, 11A, www.usatoday.com/print edition/news/20080325/oplede15.art.htm (January 7, 2011).

10. Nanci Hellmich, "Obesity Can Trim 10 Years Off Life," *USA Today*, March 18, 2009, 7D, www.usatoday.com/ news/health/weightloss/2009-03-17-obesity-death_N .htm (January 7, 2011).

11. Told to me in a phone interview.

12. Cited in Nanci Hellmich, "Obese Have Heftier Medi- cal Bills despite Shortened Lives," *USA Today*, June 10, 2008, 6D, www.usatoday.com/news/health/ weightloss/2008-06-09-obese-medical-costs_N.htm (January 7, 2011).

13. Associated Press, "Researchers Calculate the Real Cost of Being Obese," *USA Today*, September 22, 2010, 6D,

www.usatoday.com/printedition/life/20100922/hnb22
_st.art.htm (January 7, 2011).

14. Cited in Hellmich, "Obesity Can Trim 10 Years Off Life," 7D.

15. Ralph Venning, *The Sinfulness of Sin* (1669; repr., Carlisle, Pa.: Banner of Truth, 1997), 176.

16. Cited in John Carlin, "The Full Nelson," *Sports Illustrated*, August 18, 2008, 20, http://sportsillustrated.cnn.com/vault/article/magazine/MAG1143996/index.htm (January 7, 2011).

CHAPTER 10: Muscular Christianity

1. Quoted in Clifford Putney, *Muscular Christianity: Manhood and Sports in Protestant America, 1880–1920* (Cambridge, Mass.: Harvard University Press, 2001), 1.

2. Ibid., 48.

3. Ibid., 144.

4. See Tony Ladd and James Mathisen, *Muscular Christianity: Evangelical Protestants and the Development of American Sport* (Grand Rapids: Baker, 1999), 71.

5. Quoted in Putney, *Muscular Christianity*, 30.

6. Ibid., 39.

7. Ibid., 41.

8. Ibid., 50.

9. Ibid., 75.

10. Gordon Fee, *The First Epistle to the Corinthians* (Grand Rapids: Eerdmans, 1987), 94. To be fair, this quote from Fee is referencing 2:4–5, but since these verses immediately follow the passage in question and are part of the

same discussion, I believe Dr. Fee would see this as a reasonable summation of the earlier verses as well.

11. Quoted in Putney, *Muscular Christianity*, 77.

12. Ibid., 116–17.

CHAPTER 12: Stronger Shoulders

1. Kristin's quotes are taken from two sources: a personal interview with the author in March 2009 and quotations from her book *Happily Ever After* (New York: FaithWords, 2008).

2. Kristin Armstrong, *Happily Ever After: Walking with Peace and Courage Through a Year of Divorce* (New York: FaithWords, 2008), 159.

CHAPTER 13: Purely Practical

1. Dr. Kenneth H. Cooper, *Faith-Based Fitness* (Nashville: Nelson, 1995), 34.

2. Ibid., 181.

3. Ibid.

4. Quoted in Benjamin Cheever, *Strides: Running through History with an Unlikely Athlete* (New York: Rodale, 2007), 71.

5. Ibid., 72.

6. Cited in ibid., 192.

7. Quoted in ibid., 177.

8. George L. Blackburn with Julie Corliss, *Break Through Your Set Point: How to Finally Lose the Weight You Want and Keep It Off* (New York: HarperCollins, 2008).

CHAPTER 14: **Meet My Friend Morty**

1. Richard Rolle, *The English Writings*, trans. Rosamund Allen (New York: Paulist, 1988), 69.

2. John Baillie, *A Diary of Private Prayer* (New York: Scribner, 1949), 17.

3. Ibid., 35.

4. Gary Thomas, *Pure Pleasure* (Grand Rapids: Zondervan, 2009).

5. Jim Ryun, *The Courage to Run: Inspiration for Winning the Race of Your Life* (Ventura, Calif.: Regal, 2008), 118.

6. Ibid., 97.

CHAPTER 15: **The Last Christian**

1. Lorenzo Scupoli, *The Spiritual Combat* (Manchester, N.H.: Sophia Institute, 2002), 106.

2. Johannes Tauler, *Sermons*, trans. Maria Shrady (New York: Paulist, 1985), 90.

Epilogue

1. Henry Drummond, *The Ideal Life and Other Unpublished Addresses* (1899; repr., New York: Kessinger, 2003), 299.

2. Theodore Roosevelt, *The Wisdom of Theodore Roosevelt*, ed. Donald J. Davidson (New York: Citadel, 2003), 48.

3. Dean Karnazes, *Ultramarathon Man: Confessions of an All-Night Runner* (New York: Penguin, 2005), 263.

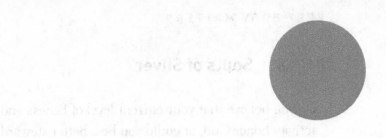

QUESTIONS FOR DISCUSSION AND REFLECTION

CHAPTER 1: **Souls of Silver**

1. Do you believe that your current level of fitness and activity honor God, or could you be a better steward in this area? What has been your biggest struggle in recent years in this regard?

2. Why do you think the church has been so silent in addressing the sins of gluttony and sloth? What are the consequences of this silence? Are there potential dangers of breaking this silence? If so, how can these dangers be guarded against?

3. Which of these elements of 2 Timothy 2:20–21 speak most directly to you?

    • becoming an instrument for special purposes

    • being made holy

    • becoming more useful to the Master

    • being prepared to do any good work

   As you think about your spiritual journey along the lines of this grid, which elements have been difficult to envision in your life?

4. Gary talks about treating our bodies like *instruments* instead of *ornaments*. How might viewing our bodies as instruments change our motivation to get in shape? How might it affect the way we evaluate our current physical condition?

5. Gary states, "Christians who don't take their health seriously don't take their mission seriously." What can you learn from having heard of someone whose ministry has been cut short due to health problems exacerbated by a soft lifestyle?

CHAPTER 2: **Heads without Bodies**

1. Have you ever done what *Christianity Today* columnist Carolyn Arends wrote about: "spiritualizing" a
   tendency toward avoiding physical fitness by focusing on "soul things" instead of "body things?" How
   can Christians keep these two arenas of stewardship
   in appropriate balance?

2. Have you ever noticed, as Karen did, a connection
   between your spiritual discipline and physical discipline? How so? Reflect on how this connection
   might be experienced in your life in everyday ways.

3. Can you pinpoint other "soul" issues that could be
   helped by focusing on physical fitness? How often
   do you hear of pastors and counselors suggesting
   that physical fitness can help in the process of healing and recovery?

4. Reread 2 Corinthians 7:1: "Dear friends, let us
   purify ourselves from everything that contaminates
   body and spirit, perfecting holiness out of reverence
   for God." Correct doctrine (what we believe) is an
   essential component of true faith, but what does this
   verse teach us about how our commitment to Christ
   calls us to something beyond that?

5. The apostle Paul in 1 Corinthians 6:20 tells us to "honor God with [our] bodies," but in 1 Thessalonians 4:4, he seems to suggest this isn't something we do naturally: "Each of you should learn to control your own body in a way that is holy and honorable." How might this "learning" be experienced in your life?

6. Karen says, "People want to hear about grace and about how much God loves them, about how they're good enough just as they are. There's a lot of truth in that, but the message about weight in our churches is that it's rude to say to someone that they need to lose weight—so we just don't address it." Do you agree that this is the current trend? What do you think of it? What would an ideal approach or response toward these issues look like?

CHAPTER 3: "Your Strength Will Equal Your Days"

1. Given your current trajectory—how your body is doing in relation to your current age—would you anticipate a vigorous or a debilitating season in your senior years? Evaluate your health habits in terms of how they might be contributing to disability or how they might be laying the foundation for many fruitful years of ministry.

2. Have you ever considered how the struggles you face in eating and exercise could be spiritual in origin, representing perhaps an attack by Satan himself? How might this understanding affect the way you address these issues?

3. Read 1 Corinthians 12:4–31. What does this passage teach about one of the themes of this book—the truth that *every body matters*? Do you believe that your ministry matters, even if you haven't identified it? How might this understanding change your motivation to exercise or to become more self-disciplined about food?

4. Read 1 Corinthians 6:19–20. Who owns your body? Give some examples of how you might treat your body when you truly believe that it belongs to God.

5. Discuss the differences between the *therapeutic* model of body care and the *stewardship* model of body care (pages 47–48). Which models do you see operating within the church?

6. Do you agree with Dr. Yphantides that, in many cases, "being unhealthy is being selfish and being healthy is being loving"? Why or why not? Bear in mind, of course, that in context, Dr. Yphantides is not addressing diseases that result from genetic factors or are not caused by poor health choices.

CHAPTER 4: **Healthy Humiliation**

1. Do you come from a Christian tradition that formally or informally ranks sins? Where is "body care" on the list of negatives? Do you think this ranking is biblically appropriate?

2. Do you agree that it's more helpful to look at overeating and sloth as a matter of remaining sensitive to God's presence rather than comparing them with lust or gossip or other sins? Why or why not?

3. Describe your history with hunger. Is it something you ever think about? Something you fear? Do you have a past that makes you particularly vulnerable to hunger? Did you pick up any insights in this chapter that will help you look at hunger in a new light?

4. Gary mentions that addressing gluttony and sloth have given him a deeper empathy for people who struggle with other sins. Did this surprise you? How well do you think the contemporary church is doing with regard to empathy for the sin struggles that others face?

CHAPTER 5: It's Not a Fair Fight

1. Read Romans 12:1. How does offering our *physical* bodies become a *spiritual* act of worship? How might Paul's words that our bodies are "holy and pleasing to God" affect the way Christians view their bodies?

2. Were you familiar with the way producers manufacture and then market food to consumers? What can the church do, if anything, to help its members come up with appropriate responses to such an assault?

3. Discuss some ways that a parent or leader could face up to their own lack of discipline in these areas, particularly in ways that will inspire others to also consider it.

4. How can the church address gluttony and sloth "through the lens of encouragement instead of judgment" and with "inspiration instead of condemnation"?

CHAPTER 6: **Is Being Overweight a Sin?**

1. Review the scriptural evidence Gary presents in this chapter and discuss the title question: Given what the Bible says and doesn't say, do you believe it is a sin to be overweight?

2. Have you noticed, as the ancients suggest, that giving in to food-related indulgence makes us weaker spiritually in the face of other temptations? How has this been evident in your own life?

3. How can Christians strike a balance, guarding against the soul becoming "accustomed to unfaithfulness" by "the neglect of little things" without being overly obsessive or pietistic about performance-based morality?

4. Is your relationship with food serving your needs physically or holding you back spiritually? How might it be a mixture of both?

5. How might affluence, including living with an abundance of food always at hand, become a threat to living a spiritually aware life?

CHAPTER 7: Socially Contagious

1. Have you ever experienced the influence of "social contagion"—either to encourage you to lose weight or to feel comfortable gaining it? What kind of environment would you say you're in now?

2. On a personal level, have you ever "decorated your chains" instead of confronting the underlying issues? Is there a physical health issue that new habits might affect, but you've just accepted it instead? What do you think might help you take action?

3. Are you primarily surrounded by people who merely accept you or by people who inspire you? Do you think you need to build a different base of support? How can Christians learn to both accept and inspire each other?

4. Discuss some ways that Christians can build health-reinforcing communities of faith. What would church look like? How might small groups spend their time differently? What kind of activities would take place?

CHAPTER 8: The Silent Murderer

1. Gary writes, "Neglect and laziness kill the best things in life." Could you list any casualties in your personal history — things and relationships that have been harmed by sloth? If you could go back in time, what would you tell yourself, knowing what you know now?

2. What area of your life is most characterized by laziness or neglect? How is it manifesting itself?

3. What kind of spiritual work has God called you to in this season of your life? Do you expect it be easy? Do you resent it when it gets hard? How do you reconcile this with Jesus' words in Matthew 11:28 telling us that he will give us rest?

4. Read 2 Timothy 2:6. What comparisons can you make between farming and Christian maturity? Are there any lessons to learn and to apply to your life?

5. Read 2 Timothy 2:15. Have you ever considered yourself a Christian "worker"? What does this verse tell you about how the apostle Paul views discipleship?

CHAPTER 9: **Let's Get Physical**

1. From a stewardship perspective, how important is it to consider how exercise can help us avoid or delay frailty? Is this end goal worthy of the amount of time consumed exercising?

2. Is it a proper motivation for Christians to pursue fitness because it makes them "feel better"? Why or why not.

3. Dr. Van Lue deals with certain issues, such as a contentious relationship between a father and a son, not just from the perspective of sin but also the perspective of physiology. Should pastors and church leaders get involved in this? Is it appropriate for Christians to consider exercise and weight loss to help treat the symptoms of depression, rage, stress, and the like?

4. Gary talks about "being kind to our bodies" by giving them sufficient exercise and better foods. How kind are you toward your body? On a scale of 1 to 10, with 1 being downright cruel and 10 being as conscientious as a person can be, how would you rate yourself?

CHAPTER 10: Muscular Christianity

1. Do the early Calvinists, who often denounced "artificial exercise" as an immoral waste of time and a sinful diversion, raise a valid issue? At what point, for instance (if ever), might it become irresponsible to train for a marathon, triathlon, or long-distance bike race?

2. To what extent should the contemporary church take up the call of Mary Dunn, who urged young people to develop bodies capable of any service God might call them to. Seminaries and Bible colleges stress doctrine and scholarship. Might it make sense for them to add some kind of focus on physical development? What benefit might this reap?

3. In what ways can competing in sports help prepare young people to work together in ministry and successfully engage in spiritual warfare?

4. Do you believe that today's church teaches a "strenuous life" in a way that can capture the imagination and interest of young people? If not, how can this be remedied, or should it become a theme worth pursuing?

5. How can a church uphold the scriptural truth that God loves and uses the weak while also calling its people to become strong?

CHAPTER 11: The Three-Hundred-Pound Pastor

1. With Karen (chapter 2) and now Mark, two individuals have testified that getting in shape not only boosted their confidence but actually improved their relationship with God. Why do you think this might be so?

2. As a youth pastor, Mark is naturally concerned about kids, particularly those who because of their age or athletic involvement may not be gaining weight, even though their eating habits are unhealthy. Along with teaching young people about spiritual matters, is there a place for youth groups to address appropriate body care? How do you think this could be done?

3. Does it surprise you that not a single Christian approached Mark about his weight? Would you talk to someone you knew was struggling with alcohol? If so, would you have a similar conversation if they were obviously hurting themselves with food? Why do you think there are "interventions" for one but not the other? What are the differences between these two struggles, and how should churches handle them differently, if at all?

4. Describe a church that excels in love. How will it balance affirmation and challenge? How will it preach unconditional acceptance while also calling people to turn from their sins and destructive habits?

5. Do you have a tendency to be more concerned about what people think about you than about their relationship with the Lord? Have you ever thought of how this is a manifestation of pride? In what other ways might pride hold us back from speaking the truth in love?

CHAPTER 12: **Stronger Shoulders**

1. Kristin came to the realization that her friends were correct in thinking that physical fitness could make her soul stronger to face the emotional challenges of a divorce and single parenting. Do you buy this? If so, how do you think it works?

2. Have you ever heard a sermon or read a book on the importance of endurance? If not, why do you think we don't talk about it more? If so, what did you learn about the place of endurance in a faithful life?

3. Have you ever heard anyone other than Kristin talk about being a "sinewy" Christian? What did you learn from her description?

4. What is the difference between using exercise to run *away from* something and using exercise to run *to* something? What are the hallmarks of a genuine "faith-based fitness?"

5. When is the last time you thought about maintaining your body as the sanctuary of the Holy Spirit? How might this thought provide new motivation?

CHAPTER 13: Purely Practical

1. Dr. Kenneth Cooper lists three elements of general fitness. Explain which one you're strongest in and which one is your weakest point:
   - regular, moderate endurance exercise
   - strength and flexibility training
   - low-fat, high-fiber diet

2. What is your favorite form of cardiovascular exercise? What might help you be more faithful in doing this?

3. Do you have any routines that might be impairing your health? Discuss some strategies to break out of a particularly troublesome routine.

4. Do you think you would be more faithful exercising if you had some exercise partners? Talk about ways you can build such a support group.

5. Discuss the importance of grace and gentleness for those who embark on a new fitness program.

CHAPTER 14: Meet My Friend Morty

1. How faithful are we in general—and you in particular—to obey Paul's words to Timothy to actively "pursue righteousness, godliness, faith, love, endurance and gentleness"? What excuses do we give? Did you grow up in a theological tradition that might even question the need for this? How does your current faith community help you meet the challenge of 1 Timothy 6:11?

2. Has your belief in what is possible—overcoming a particular sin or habit—been shaped more by your experience of past failure or by God's Word? How can we sustain the courage to keep up the pursuit when we've failed so many times before?

3. Gary writes that "every point of sin is a point of disagreement with God. And when we disagree with God, guess who is in the wrong?" What disagreements do you have with God about eating, exercise, and overall fitness? How can thinking this through better prepare you for the next time? As Gary points out, "At least make Satan come up with a new lie!"

4. Review the acts of mortification:

   - Taste the bitterness of your sin

   - Examine the deceit behind the sin.

   - Consider the circumstances of your sin.

   - Use the exposure that sin provides to gain a more accurate view of the condition of your soul.

   - Consider the strength of your sin.

   - Find a holy substitute.

   - Fortify your soul.

   Have you ever responded to sin this thoughtfully? Did any one of these strike you as being more helpful to you in particular?

5. Read 1 Corinthians 9:24–27; 2 Timothy 4:5–8; and Hebrews 12:1–2. Gary writes of Boston, "If the pursuit had been easy, there wouldn't have been half the joy in finishing the race." Do you think life is somewhat like that? What light do the above Scriptures shed on this?

CHAPTER 15: The Last Christian

1. Do you agree that the church today needs to "get tougher"? Why or why not?

2. We live during a time when many Christians assume that life in Christ leads to an easier life rather than a more troublesome one. Do you think it's possible for a Christian today to pray as Jeremiah did, with "pain unending, wounds grievous and incurable"?

3. How can the church help prepare its members for times of testing, persecution, and challenge? Do you think it's appropriate to consider physical fitness as an ingredient in this preparation? Why or why not?

4. Given all that you've read, describe your thoughts on the motivation for, the importance of, and the depth of your conviction to practice increased physical fitness.

GARY THOMAS

Feel free to contact Gary at glt3@aol.com. Though he cannot respond personally to all correspondence, he would love to get your feedback. Please understand, however, that he is neither qualified nor able to provide counsel via e-mail.

For information about Gary's speaking schedule, visit his website (www.garythomas.com). Follow him on Twitter (garyLthomas) or connect with him on Facebook. To inquire about inviting Gary to your church, please e-mail his assistant: laura@garythomas.com.

Simply Sacred

Daily Readings

Gary Thomas

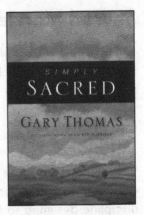

Gary Thomas is a popular writer of Christian spirituality with a well-developed platform.

Building on his bestselling books *Sacred Pathways* and *Sacred Marriage*; his newest book, *Pure Pleasure*; and his Gold Medallion-winning *Authentic Faith*, Thomas takes readers to new levels of inspiration and insight in *Simply Sacred*—a devotional made up of selections from his best writings about spirituality and spiritual formation.

According to Thomas, "Those who have advanced in the Christian life have learned to develop an almost mystical memory that keeps them attuned to the fact that God is always with them ... always watching, always caring, always hearing."

Abounding with spiritual insights and practical truth, this book provides readers with the freedom to approach life in Christ with new wonder and joy each and every day.

Available in stores and online!

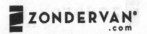

Sacred Marriage

What If God Designed Marriage to Make Us Holy More Than to Make Us Happy?

Gary Thomas

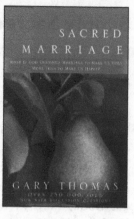

Your marriage is more than a sacred covenant with another person. It is a spiritual discipline designed to help you know God better, trust him more fully, and love him more deeply.

Scores of books have been written that offer guidance for building the marriage of your dreams. But what if God's primary intent for your marriage isn't to make you happy — but holy? And what if your relationship isn't as much about you and your spouse as it is about you and God?

Everything about your marriage is filled with prophetic potential, with the capacity for discovering and revealing Christ's character. The respect you accord your partner; the forgiveness you humbly seek and graciously extend; the ecstasy, awe, and sheer fun of lovemaking; the history you and your spouse build with each other — in these and other facets of your marriage, *Sacred Marriage* uncovers the mystery of God's overarching purpose.

This book may well alter profoundly the contours of your marriage. It will most certainly change you. Because whether it is delightful or difficult, your marriage can become a doorway to a closer walk with God and to a spiritual integrity that, like salt, seasons the world around you with the savor of Christ.

Available in stores and online!

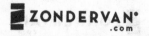

ZONDERVAN®
.com

Sacred Marriage Gift Edition

Gary Thomas

This special edition two-in-one book and devotional includes:

Sacred Marriage

Starting with the discovery that the goal of marriage goes beyond personal happiness, writer and speaker Gary Thomas invites readers to see how God can use marriage as a discipline and a motivation to love him more and reflect more of the character of his Son.

Devotions for a Sacred Marriage

A companion to *Sacred Marriage*, these fifty-two devotions encourage you to build your marriage around God's priorities. From learning to live with a fellow sinner, to the process of two becoming one, to sharing our lives as brothers and sisters in Christ, *Devotions for a Sacred Marriage* challenges couples to embrace the profound and soul-stretching reality of Christian marriage.

Available in stores and online!

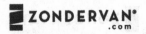

ZONDERVAN®
.com

Sacred Pathways

Discover Your Soul's Path to God

Gary Thomas, Bestselling Author of Sacred Marriage

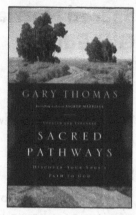

"Thou shalt not covet thy neighbor's spiritual walk." After all, it's his, not yours. Better to discover the path God designed *you* to take—a path marked by growth and fulfillment, based on your own unique temperament.

In *Sacred Pathways*, Gary Thomas strips away the frustration of a one-size-fits-all spirituality and guides you toward a path of worship that frees you to be you. If your devotional times have hit a snag, perhaps it's because you're trying to follow someone else's path.

This book unpacks nine distinct spiritual temperaments—their traits, strengths, and pitfalls. In one or more of them, you will see yourself and the ways you most naturally express your relationship with Jesus Christ. Whatever temperament or blend of temperaments best describes you, rest assured it's not by accident. It's by the design of a Creator who knew what he was doing when he made you according to his own unique specifications. *Sacred Pathways* will reveal the route you were made to travel, marked by growth and filled with the riches of a close walk with God.

Available in stores and online!

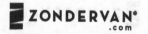

ZONDERVAN®
.com

Sacred Parenting

How Raising Children Shapes Our Souls

Gary Thomas

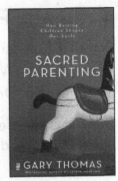

Many books have been written about how to parent a child effectively, how to become a better parent, and how effective parenting produces better kids. But *Sacred Parenting* delves into a different reality: how parenting affects the parent. It explores the spiritual dynamics of parenting, and why caring for children is such an effective discipline in shaping our souls and forming the character of Christ within us. Parents of all children will be encouraged by seeing how others have successfully handled the challenges of parenting and will be inspired by stories that reaffirm the spiritual value of being a parent.

Devotions for Sacred Parenting

A Year of Weekly Devotions for Parents

Gary Thomas

Spend time once a week for an entire year contemplating the soul-transforming journey of parenting.

Devotions for Sacred Parenting continues this journey with fifty-two short devotions, containing all new material. The life-related devotions are creative and fresh, and readers will be inspired, challenged, and encouraged as they explore the spiritual joys and challenges of raising children. Each devotion will point them to opportunities for spiritual growth — and help them become more effective parents at the same time.

Authentic Faith

What If Life Isn't Meant to Be Perfect, but We Are Meant to Trust the One Who Is?

Gary Thomas, Bestselling Author of Sacred Marriage

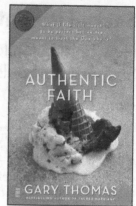

What if the spiritual disciplines that bring us closer to God are not the ones we control? Bestselling author Gary Thomas reveals the rich benefits that derive from embracing the harder truths of Scripture. With penetrating insight from Scripture and the Christian classics, along with colorful and engaging stories, Thomas's eye-opening look into what it means to be a true disciple of Jesus will encourage you, bolster your faith, and help you rise above shallow attachments to fix your heart on things of eternal worth.

Thomas shows us that authentic faith penetrates the most unlikely places. It is found when we die to ourselves and put others first. It is nurtured when we cultivate contentment instead of spending our energy trying to improve our lot in life. It is strengthened in suffering, persecution, waiting, and even mourning. Instead of holding on to grudges, authentic faith chooses forgiveness. And it lives with another world in mind, recognizing that what we do in this broken world will be judged.

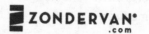

Holy Available

What If Holiness Is about More Than What We Don't Do?

Gary Thomas, Bestselling author of Sacred Marriage

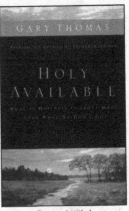

Previously titled
The Beautiful Fight

True Christian faith is a profoundly transformational experience in which every part of our being is marked by God's change and energized by his presence. This transformation takes us far beyond mere sin avoidance to a robust, "full-bodied" holiness in which we make ourselves "holy available" to God every minute of the day. From Starbucks, to the office, to the soccer fields, to the boardroom, believers have the opportunity to carry the presence of Christ wherever they go.

God offers the reader more than mere forgiveness; he wants to radically change and fill them with his presence, so they can experience an entirely different kind of life based not just on what they do or don't do but on who they are.

Yet while many Christians today profess belief, their Christianity has no pulse. Previously titled *The Beautiful Fight*, *Holy Available* is a manifesto of fully alive faith. Gary Thomas issues a compelling call for readers to see with Christ's eyes, feel with Christ's heart, and serve with Christ's hands. We make ourselves available to become "God oases," places of spiritual refuge where God can bring the hurting and lost to enjoy his presence and ministry.

Available in stores and online!

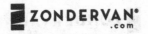

Pure Pleasure

Why Do Christians Feel So Bad about Feeling Good?

Gary Thomas, Bestselling Author of Sacred Marriage

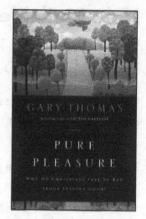

Discover the power of guilt-free pleasure.

Pleasure is a good thing. It's a powerful force that feeds your relationships, helps protect your spiritual integrity, and brings delight to our heavenly Father. Pleasure isn't something Christians should fear, shun, or disparage; it's something we should learn to cultivate in our lives.

Acclaimed spiritual growth author Gary Thomas will guide you into this way of life, which is foundational to a healthy relationship with God, with your loved ones, and with the world. He'll show you that, for the redeemed, pleasure can be a powerful and holy force for good, leading to increased worship, spiritual strength, and renewed relationships.

In this invigorating and liberating book, Gary Thomas will energize, inspire, equip, and challenge you to experience life as God meant it to be: overflowing with pleasure.

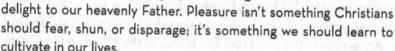

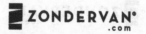

Share Your Thoughts

With the Author: Your comments will be forwarded to the author when you send them to *zauthor@zondervan.com*.

With Zondervan: Submit your review of this book by writing to *zreview@zondervan.com*.

Free Online Resources at
www.zondervan.com

Zondervan AuthorTracker: Be notified whenever your favorite authors publish new books, go on tour, or post an update about what's happening in their lives at www.zondervan.com/authortracker.

Daily Bible Verses and Devotions: Enrich your life with daily Bible verses or devotions that help you start every morning focused on God. Visit www.zondervan.com/newsletters.

Free Email Publications: Sign up for newsletters on Christian living, academic resources, church ministry, fiction, children's resources, and more. Visit www.zondervan.com/newsletters.

Zondervan Bible Search: Find and compare Bible passages in a variety of translations at www.zondervanbiblesearch.com.

Other Benefits: Register to receive online benefits like coupons and special offers, or to participate in research.

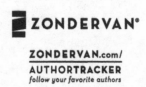

ZONDERVAN

ZONDERVAN.com/
AUTHORTRACKER
follow your favorite authors